D1536740

5 CHANGE MANAGEMENT STRATEGIES TO TRANSFORM YOUR HEALTH

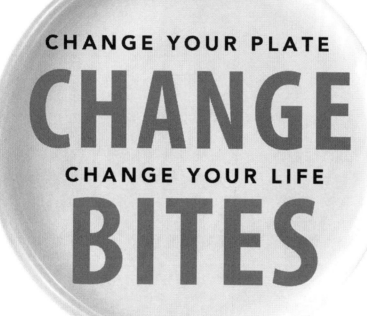

CHANGE YOUR PLATE

CHANGE

CHANGE YOUR LIFE

BITES

WRITTEN BY

MARISSA S. COSTONIS, H.C.

Change Bites, 5 Change Management Strategies to Transform Your Health.
Copyright © 2018 by Marissa Costonis All rights reserved.

ISBN-13: 978-0-692-11377-6
Library of Congress Control Number: 2018905816

Printed in the United States of America

CONTENTS

Introduction

I can't remember the first time I felt the numbness and tingling sensation go up and down my leg like a giant wave, but I do remember standing in the kitchen, cooking for a big family picnic, wondering why my nerves were now firing over thirty times a day. I literally shook it off. But after a few months and a few Google searches later, I knew my body was desperately trying to communicate with me. I just didn't understand the language.

At its peak, this "neuropathy" (nerve pain, numbness, and tingling) spread from my left leg to my right leg, then up both arms, and on bad days, to my face. Surprise, shock, and utter fear took over and I knew I couldn't ignore it any longer. As a young mother of two, with a husband who traveled a lot for work, there was no time to be sick. I thought, *How is it possible that I am the picture of health on the outside and a complete mess on the inside?* Ironically, my doctor had recently told me at my annual well-visit that he wished all his patients were as "healthy" as me. Thank God they weren't.

I began to wonder what else my body had tried to tell me over the years? I brushed off several health problems, including chronic sinus and viral infections, which left me in bed for weeks, a lifelong battle with constipation, migraines, congestion, excessive fatigue, high white blood cell count, and an episode of Bell's palsy (facial paralysis on one side) to name a few. *Could all these symptoms be connected in some way?* Like it or not, I needed to take the time and find out, right then.

Traditional medicine seemed to be a good place to start. My primary care physician and neurologist ordered a battery of tests, which all came back negative. So, I was sent off to figure this out on my own. Three frustrating years of appointments and a variety of treatments with countless doctors, specialists, and wellness practitioners yielded marginal success. I was convinced that multiple sclerosis or some other autoimmune disease or cancer was imminent. Paranoid that I would get every common cold or virus, I developed some OCD behaviors to keep the germs away. After a family party, I found myself cleaning doorknobs, toilet handles, and light switches, determined to stay healthy. I became obsessed by my symptoms and fell for every possible treatment available. As supportive as they were, the glazed look on my family's and friend's faces told me that their patience was waning, and so was mine.

One night, my sister dragged me to a party with a guest psychic for fun. When my turn came to ask a question, I said in frustration and fear, "Am I going to find answers and am I going to be okay?" It felt as if she stared through to my soul and responded with confidence, "Yes, Marissa, you are going to be fine and will get some answers soon." She could have been the Wizard of Oz for all I know, but she gave me motivation to keep plugging along.

A few months later, I was thrilled to finally find someone who had some concrete answers. He told me that my metal levels were through the roof, my immune system was still weak from the mononucleosis I had as a child (the Epstein-Barr virus), and that my gut was almost completely void of any "good" bacteria from years of antibiotic overuse. He concurred that this health problem could turn into something much more severe if not addressed. With some answers in hand, I was ready to get started with a plan. Of course, as in the past, I was expecting some pill, spray, powder, or other prescription for health, but what I got was something way worse. He told me I had to completely change my diet. Apparently, the power of my healing started on my plate.

While I should have been relieved, I walked out of the doctor's office in tears, completely overwhelmed by the idea of needing to fundamentally change everything I knew about food. Being 100% Italian-American, my eating habits, cooking methods, and food traditions are at the heart of who I am. He wanted me to give up dairy and all grains, including pasta, bread, and pizza. What's left after taking all that out?

With over 100 diet plans available outlining WHAT to eat and what not to eat, I couldn't find much information on HOW to begin changing my lifelong eating habits. All I could find were BEFORE and AFTER pictures and glamorized stories of health transformations, but rarely did I see the struggle in between the two. **Managing the change and the transition to**

a new way of eating was the missing piece. This was going to be the real challenge.

The concept of change was not new to me. I spent over a decade in a specialized form of management consulting called "change management." My job was to ensure that employees embraced proposed business changes and that the transition to the new solution was a smooth one. I have helped plan mergers, structure new organization models, performance measurement systems, and countless process designs. For someone who spent more than a decade helping Fortune 500 companies around the world through all kinds of change, the simple idea of changing my diet and giving up the foods I loved left me paralyzed.

After assessing my situation, I began to wonder if any of the change management frameworks I had used with great success in business could apply to my own personal food and health transformation. So, I went back to all the books, models, and best practices, and began to put the pieces together. If 90% of corporate change initiatives are deemed a success today[1] and 95% of all diets reportedly fail[2], surely there is something to be learned from businesses and change.

Using myself as a guinea pig, I began to create a new health change model and **The 5 Bites to Health was born!** My "go slow to go fast" approach—used so many times in business—was the missing piece to transitioning to a new way of eating, one bite at a time. This approach acknowledges the difficulty of change, values careful planning, and supports gradual changes that are sustainable over time. An individual aiming for "perfect" health and a corporation striving to increase profits both have the same goal. They both embark upon change to maximize benefits and hopefully realize them sooner than later.

I experienced many struggles and successes in my food transition. In fact, my symptoms became a lot worse before they got better. But with determination, I persevered and finally began to see results. Today, I am happier and healthier than ever.

Upon embarking on my health journey, what I didn't realize was just how much better I would feel in so many other aspects of my health. As the tingling and numbness throughout my body subsided, I also experienced significant improvements in my digestion, sinuses, energy, skin appearance, and sleep. As it turns out, I had a severe gluten and dairy intolerance my whole life! The transformation process even had a positive effect on my family's health as they, too, identified several unknown food intolerances. Now, they are armed with the knowledge and skills to make completely different food choices to keep themselves healthy. It's true that you don't know how sick you are until you get better!

Inspired by my own health transformation, I decided to take my change skills to the next level and attend the Institute for Integrative Nutrition in New York and become a certified health coach. I now use my background in change management with my training in nutrition to guide others in their own journey to health. Managing my own health challenges and working with my health coaching clients allowed me to fine tune The 5 Bites to Health with great results.

Do you want to change how you eat to improve your health? Perhaps you received a diagnosis, have an allergy, or are simply fed up with a growing list of symptoms and have decided enough is enough. Maybe you were inspired by a new book or documentary to try a new diet but could use a little help with the transition. No matter how good or bad your diet is today, we can all stand to make a few improvements. **Allow me to be your personal change management consultant and let this book guide you in your own personal health journey!** Learn from my mistakes and know that I won't pretend that change is easy but rather provide you with much needed structure and support along the way.

In this book, I will share stories from my personal transition, business transformation examples, as well as real health coaching stories to show you that all change is relatable. I hope that you will find yourself somewhere in these examples and can use them to support your own transition. You will notice that communication is a critical component in each of the five steps of the model. Communication and support are key to a successful business change and your transformation is almost impossible without them.

Throughout the book, I will also ask you to stop and "savor" each bite. This represents the time needed to stop and reflect honestly about how the change is going so you can adjust your plan accordingly. Remember, this isn't a race, so get to the finish line at your own pace. It doesn't matter where you start from or how long it takes to get there. The goal is to keep moving forward and making progress.

To gather additional data, I conducted a food transition survey with over 100 people who have a health problem that may be impacted by changes in their diet. **85% of responders reported that changes in their diet helped their symptoms or contributed to their healing.** Data on what contributed and hindered their transition to a new way of eating was quite insightful. I will share additional details of the survey throughout the book so you, too, can learn from their experiences.

You are provided with a variety of tools to reflect, journal, and create a specific plan of action to support your own transition. You can request additional copies of the tools, worksheets, questions, and activities on my website (ChangeBites.com). Trust the change process and I promise we will get through this together.

Change is difficult. Change is messy. Change BITES! This book acknowledges the struggles of change, but also provides you with practical tips to guide you in your journey to health. You will learn to interpret the sounds of your body's cries and will know exactly what it needs for comfort. I promise you will end up on the other side of change in a dramatically better place, both physically and mentally. Change will become your new favorite habit. After it's over, you may just find yourself wondering what all the fuss was about in the first place.

CHAPTER ONE

What's Your Health Story?

The word "health" is so overused and it varies greatly from one person to the next. If you are considering a change in your eating habits to improve your health, it's important to take some time to determine what "health" means to you. To properly define "health," we must first go backwards just a bit and begin to assemble your personal health story. This is the first example of my "go slow to go fast" approach. Trust me, taking the time to understand how you got to this point in your life and your health is key before setting out to change it.

So many people today have a health story that reads more like a novel. At least 50 million Americans suffer from over 100 autoimmune diseases (that's 1 in 5 people).[3] These diseases are often hard to diagnose, leaving many to manage their symptoms for years before getting any answers or relief. More than 100 million people in the United States have diabetes or prediabetes[4], and more than 1 in 3 children in the U.S. have allergic diseases such as food allergies, asthma, and eczema.[5] No matter how you slice the statistics, the overall health story in the U.S. today is not a pretty picture. Many illnesses seem to pop up out of nowhere, but many have built up over a lifetime. Therefore, it is so important that we begin to put the pieces of our health together and find a pattern in our story.

Perhaps the culprit and the cure is in our food. I knew that 80% of our immune system lives in our gastrointestinal tract[6], but I was surprised to learn from the food transition survey that **85% of people said they followed some dietary restrictions to improve their symptoms/condition (i.e. gluten-free, vegan, low sugar, paleo, dairy-free, etc.).** Not only are we finally recognizing that food can make a huge difference in our health and healing, we are starting to change!

Ironically, we haven't seen a lot of data around diet and prevention of disease until recently. However, the latest report indicates that 45% percent of all deaths (over 700,000) from heart disease, stroke, and diabetes could be prevented by changes in diet.[7] The report goes on to recommend that we need to eat more foods that are good for us (i.e. real whole foods) and less foods that are bad for us (i.e. processed, packaged foods). Shocking to think that this is startling new research!

PERSONAL BITE

Before my neuropathy, I never thought of my health as one complete story. In fact, I didn't even realize that I had one to tell. I thought of my health in compartments versus one complete picture. I went to a gastroenterologist for my digestive problems, my primary care physician for strep throat or other infections, an ENT (Ears, Nose, Throat) doctor for my sinus issues, a neurologist for my nerve pain, and so on. Using this model often left me on my own for other health problems such as insomnia, anxiety, fatigue, and the stress of being a parent, which were also key inputs to defining my current state of health.

Even my frequent illnesses as a child played a role in defining my health story. My struggle with mononucleosis at twelve left me with a low white blood cell count and highly vulnerable to sore throats and viral infections for years. This virus likely played a role in getting Bell's palsy just days before giving birth to my first son.

When I gained online access to my health records from the last ten years, I thought it was the wrong file. I couldn't remember all the visits and ailments over the years. Compiling my health history into one story gave me great perspective on how I'd arrived at my current state of health as well as some insight into how I needed to change it.

BUSINESS BITE

When consulting with a new organization faced with a challenge, we always take some time to reflect on the company's past while looking forward to the objectives they are trying to achieve. This step applies equally to a brand new startup or a company in existence for over a hundred years. We ask questions such as, "What makes this company unique in the market?" Or, "What is the company's experience with change initiatives in the past (both good and bad)?" We look at past and current data (i.e. sales, business strategy, customer service, and market share) and how it compares to the competition. We also assess the culture of the executive team as this tends to filter down the organization. Taking time to understand the history and general state of the client's business is important before developing their future solutions. Just as you have a short or long health story, so does each business embarking upon a change.

BEFORE YOU BITE

What's your health story? Is it a short story or more of a novel? Remember that your definition of "health" is comprised of more than just your physical wellbeing. The history of your stress, sleep, relationships, diet, and past illnesses are all important factors. How would you describe the quality of food in your family today and in the past?

Recognize if you and your partner or your entire family share vastly different eating styles from one another. Your parents' and extended family's health history may also be important. If every male over the age of fifty has either survived a heart attack or passed away from one, this could be an important part of your own health story.

Take some time to articulate your health story using the worksheet provided. Be honest and don't leave anything out. Try to obtain access to your medical file from your primary care physician or any specialists you have seen over the years. Don't overlook minor problems such as a little heartburn, eczema, or the occasional headache. Now is the time to acknowledge all your ailments from childhood until now to create a full picture of your health.

YOUR HEALTH STORY

Take some time to write your personal health story using the questions below.

What major/minor health challenges or symptoms have you experienced?

What are your major daily stressors?

What role does exercise play in your life?

Do you have strong relationships to keep you balanced?

Describe your current sleep patterns and digestive health?

How would you describe your diet (past/present)?

_____

_____

_____

_____

_____

_____

_____

_____

_____

_____

_____

_____

SAVOR IT: Take a step back and reflect on your health story. Are you surprised by anything? Were their things about your health you forgot about? If you handed this story to a stranger, how would they describe the health of this person?

Whether your health story reads more like a short poem or a copy of the Odyssey, it's important to review it in its entirety. We all have little health challenges that individually aren't a big deal. We take a pill or prescription here and there to address it. However, when our ailments begin to pile up and we take a step back, we are often alarmed at how long the list is. If you have uncovered a bigger health problem, take the time to search and find the root cause. Once we take the time to understand our story, we can then identify the role that food and wellness practices play in mapping out our next chapter.

CHAPTER TWO

7 Deadly Sins of Change

Grab a blank sheet of paper and sign your official full name. This is familiar, easy, and you can probably do this with your eyes closed. Now, put the pen in your opposite hand and do the same thing. The lines don't flow, the process takes a lot more concentration, and, for me, it feels like everything is in slow motion with pitiful results to show for it. This is what it feels like to change. A simple shift to the off-hand takes you right out of your comfort zone.

Change is easier said than done whether you are an individual trying to follow a new eating strategy or a business motivated to execute a new strategic plan. Based on my experience, I have identified 7 deadly sins of organization change that can also be applied to assist you in your transition to a new way of eating.

1. *No Sense of Urgency*
2. *No Clear Vision*
3. *Poor Planning*
4. *Lack of Leadership*
5. *Poor Communication/Support*
6. *Lack of Training*
7. *Fear of Failure*

1 NO SENSE OF URGENCY

Imagine you are enjoying a nice pad Thai from the new restaurant down the street, and out of nowhere, your throat starts to get itchy and you have trouble breathing. Luckily, you get to the hospital in plenty of time to get the appropriate medicine and all is well. Through this process, you discover a new peanut allergy. Your sense of urgency is high, to say the least, and your need to eliminate peanuts from your diet is obvious. There is no room for error in this scenario and every precaution must be taken from here on out to avoid peanuts in every shape and form. Everyone in the family who might cook for you must also be on board with this change to ensure your food is prepared safely.

Now, compare this to someone else who gets terrible gas, congestion, and snores all night after eating pork. The sense of urgency is a lot lower and, therefore, the need to avoid this food is a lot less critical (although much appreciated by their spouse).

Let's apply the same scenario in a business setting. A large manufacturing company is faced with rapidly declining sales and decreased market share. They need to make some major changes or face going out of business. They restructure their organization, cutting 150 jobs, and adjust their pricing and distribution strategy. A thoughtful change management plan is rolled out to employees to gain their support and quickly implement the changes and realize proposed benefits. Whether you are a business or individual, it is always easier to embrace change if you understand that the consequences of not changing are far worse.

2 NO CLEAR VISION

You must visualize the future you want to achieve. If you haven't first defined success, how do you know when you have achieved it? A clear vision helps you stay focused, minimizes frustration, and keeps you motivated throughout any change process. This is particularly helpful in a food transition. For example, giving up chocolate for a chocoholic doesn't seem as hard if you are focused on the goal of eliminating chronic migraines.

My overall vision was very clear from the beginning. I wanted to keep the neuropathy from spreading to my right leg, arms, and face, and eventually, I wanted to eliminate it from my left leg all together. I also wanted to get some relief from my chronic constipation. Yes, my vision was to live life without numbness and tingling in my legs and simply poop every day. The basic things we take for granted! Focusing on my goals kept me on track when everyone else was eating gourmet pizza and I was left with the gluten-free version or a salad. Communicating my vision clearly to those close to me also allowed them to provide me with much needed support along the way.

Employees at all levels in the organization must have a common understanding of the vision and reason for change. While this might seem to be an easy task as it is simply a function of good communication, it is a very common pitfall that inhibits successful change initiatives all the time. In fact, 95% of a company's employees are unaware of, or do not understand, its strategy.[8] If employees do not understand why the company is changing and how they can directly make a difference, it's hard for them to support it.

I once worked with an insurance company in Belgium whose goal was to move from fifth to second in their market. I helped them create a new operating model, organization structure, and a results-based claims process. They were undergoing a massive change transformation and needed support from everyone in the organization to make their vision a reality. It wasn't enough for everyone to know WHAT was changing, but they needed a clear vision for WHY it was so important. As a result, all employees understood how they fit into the new strategy and everyone was on board to support the change.

3 POOR PLANNING

It quickly became apparent that if I didn't plan ahead and keep the proper foods in my kitchen, I was going to be starving all the time. You wouldn't know it to see me, but I have a huge appetite. The more prepared I was, the easier the transition to a new way of eating became.

Lack of planning is the most common downfall I hear from my health coaching clients. This theory was also confirmed in the food transition survey. Almost 60% of respondents reported that "making time to shop and cook" (i.e. planning) was a key success factor when transitioning to a new way of eating to improve their health. You will be provided a variety of ways to simplify the food planning process throughout this book.

Proper planning for any business change is just as important. Imagine a toy company launching a new product for Christmas, but due to improper planning and scheduling, it doesn't reach shelves across the country until December 27th. It's the same as taking the time to shop and stock your refrigerator with tons of fresh produce but when 6pm rolls around you have nothing prepared for dinner. Batch cooking some staples such as quinoa or roasted veggies ahead of time can help. Be sure to plan the extra step to enjoy the rewards.

4 LACK OF LEADERSHIP

In a business transformation, strong leadership and project management are critical to motivate employees to support the change. Project tasks such as planning, tracking project performance, and recognizing success are key. Strong leaders walk the talk and make change happen, pushing through difficult obstacles along the way.

This leadership was exactly what I needed for my own transformation. Similar tasks included food planning, measuring my progress against my health goals, and recognizing my health successes along the way. I celebrated each month my neuropathy and digestion improved, and this kept me motivated. When it became very difficult to eat differently, I channeled strong leadership skills to persevere and earn the respect of others. As a true leader, I hoped to inspire someone else through my own actions to make a food change in the future.

Take initiative and don't wait for someone else to make it all happen. You are ultimately the one responsible for executing your new eating strategy and getting control of your health. You are a strong leader and can do whatever you set your mind to!

5 POOR COMMUNICATION/SUPPORT

Continued communication with all parties involved in a change is critical both in business and in health. If I was going to completely change my entire diet, I couldn't do it without letting my family and friends know what was happening and soliciting their support. My new eating style was inevitably going to impact how I cooked for my family, what restaurants we dined at, etc. It was my job to communicate the right amount of information to those close to me so they could support me along the way. The more encouragement they provided me, the better!

Maintain communication with your "tribe" of family and friends around you. They can support you if they understand your problem and specifically how to help you. For example, when going to family's or a friend's house for dinner, I always made something that I could eat and everyone could enjoy. To show their support, my tribe alters their menu a bit to ensure I don't go hungry. They may also surprise me with a special dessert that is gluten and dairy-free!

6 LACK OF TRAINING

When transitioning to a new way of eating, I had to educate myself on how to shop and cook differently to accommodate the change. A variety of books, cooking sites, and recipe blogs provided me with easy substitutions and gave me the skills and confidence I needed to keep trying new techniques.

Imagine installing drastically new technology overnight in an organization without providing any training whatsoever! Proper training (one-on-one, on-the-job, and integrated directly into the system) minimizes frustration and can help achieve benefits sooner than expected.

Let's say you were inspired to change by a new documentary about following a vegan diet and are motivated to get started immediately. Any positive change to improve your health is wonderful. However, don't forget that you too may benefit from some training. For example, adequate B12 in the form of fortified foods or supplements may be needed to support your vegan diet. Consider taking an online vegan cooking class or take a trip to your local bookstore to find a new vegan cookbook. Gaining additional knowledge can only help increase your chances for success. Any other training you can learn "on-the-job" or in the kitchen.

7 FEAR OF FAILURE

Many individuals and businesses are afraid of radical change because it often results in some failure initially. Remember when you tried to sign your name with your non-dominant hand? Of course, you weren't going to be perfect at it on your first try (unless you are ambidextrous). But if you took some time to practice, you would get pretty good at it. Don't be afraid. There is arguably more to learn from failure than success.

Businesses have no choice but to change in today's rapidly moving environment. However, some companies may be a bit hesitant to make certain changes that were tried and failed in the past. Perhaps a new product rollout was a disaster a few years ago but now, with some tweaks in design, pricing and implementation strategy, it is a huge success. Some employees may have a "been there, tried that, and it didn't work" mentality and are afraid to try again. They don't want to waste their time and energy again on a repeated failure, so they resist the change. This is the time to explain how we can learn from our mistakes to create a much better outcome.

Have you tried a bunch of eating styles in the past with little success? Maybe you tried a special recipe and it ended with a bunch of smoke and take-out? This may leave you a bit hesitant to try again. Don't let past failure get in the way of your future success. Don't let that stop you. Just keep the fire extinguisher close by and you'll be fine.

Expect some bumps on the road to changing your diet and your health. Making any big change is easier with a high sense of urgency and clear vision. Channel your inner executive skills to demonstrate strong planning and leadership. Don't expect to jump into your new eating style without any preparation at all. It's just like starting a new job. You may be a bit nervous at first, but you can't be afraid to fail. Once you get some training and practice, you'll get the hang of it in no time!

CHAPTER THREE

The 5 Bites to Health

There are many models and frameworks through which to describe how people move through the change process. One of the original change curves was created by Elizabeth Kubler-Ross in 1969 to manage the stages of grief for those surviving or approaching death. This original change model and others have been altered over the last fifty years in a variety of ways to shed some light on the complexity of change in the business world. The pace of change in business today is rapid, and companies today are arguably far more adept at change than ever before. I have found that the process of change and methods for moving through it are surprisingly similar whether you are a CEO navigating a recent merger, a mom transitioning her child's diet to address a new allergy, or an individual shifting to a vegan lifestyle. The goals are also similar in each of these scenarios: get through the change with minimal pain and disruption to enjoy all the proposed benefits as quickly as possible.

It seemed fitting to go back to a model used for the grieving process since that's exactly how I felt at the idea of giving up foods I loved. In my own personal health journey and in my experience with organizations around the world facing major change, I find that a similar set of five change management strategies or best practices hold true. With that in mind, I created a new change management model called "The 5 Bites to Health" that outlines my unique perspective and approach. The steps in this model have made all the difference in my own transformation and have led to great success with my health coaching clients as well.

Remember that The 5 Bites to Health is not a linear process. The steps are organic and the route and time frame to get through each one varies for each person. You will go back and forth and up and down between steps for weeks, months, or even years. Eventually, you will end up on the other side, in a remarkably better place.

The more adept you are at change, the more opportunities you will have in life. Change flexibility may open the door to a new hobby, career, friends, or newly found passion, no matter your age. To arm you with these important change skills, I have outlined three actions for each step in The 5 Bites to Health. This change model can be used to support a small change (i.e. reduce sugar or increase intake of leafy greens), or a transition to an entirely new way of eating (i.e. grain-free or vegan diet). You can use this model over and over to implement and build upon a variety of changes in your life.

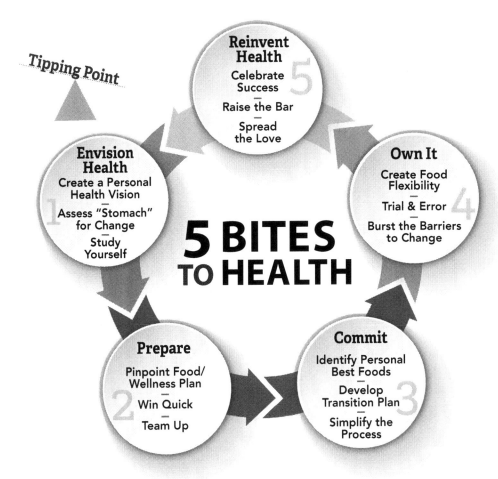

Before You Begin - The Tipping Point What sparked your interest in making a food transition and a health transformation? Did a symptom scare you out of nowhere or did your doctor shock you with a diagnosis? Perhaps it was a growing list of small ailments that put you over the edge. Maybe you were inspired to take charge of your future health by a recent book or documentary. Whatever tipped you over the edge, congratulations on taking the first step!

The "tipping point," as described by Malcolm Gladwell, is "that magic moment when an idea, trend, or social behavior crosses a threshold, tips, and spreads like wildfire."[9] We are seeing a tipping point in the area of health. Over the last few years, the rise in health-conscious menu items, restaurants, stores, and food choices is remarkable. But even with a greater sense of health awareness, the number of individuals with food-related diseases continues to rise. We need to increase this momentum to make sustainable changes to our health!

Imagine you are standing at the window of your apartment building and it is engulfed in flames, twenty stories high. You are contemplating jumping down into the net to save yourself but not sure you will survive the fall. The reality is that you have no choice but to jump because staying put isn't an option. Imagine your health is the burning apartment. With rates of disease, allergies, and food sensitivities so high, you risk going down in flames at some point if you keep doing what you're doing. If you already suffer from some sort of health problem, your desire to jump may be high. It's a lot easier to take a leap of faith if your current state of "pain" is worse than the pain of changing. What have you got to lose?

> *It's a lot easier to take a leap of faith if your current state of "pain" is worse than the pain of changing.*

Many people never reach their tipping point because they are stuck in some form of denial. They may be in denial that they have a problem, or they are in denial over the idea that changing their food can have a significant, life-altering impact on their health. It's like the person in the fire scenario doesn't believe the house is on fire, and even if they do, they aren't looking for the window yet alone the safety net down below.

Adam is a good example of denial. He lives with IBS (irritable bowel syndrome) and has a weak immune system, often leaving him sick with a virus and cold sores. His brother was diagnosed with celiac and his cousin has Crohn's disease. Adam suspects that he has some type of gluten sensitivity. He's getting married, just bought a new house, and things are hectic at work. The last thing he can handle is the chaos of changing his entire diet. He chooses to ignore the problem because he simply can't handle the change right now.

Many are in denial out of self-preservation. Some just aren't ready for the challenge at this point in their lives, and I totally get it. There are times when we can handle change and times we know we can't. I see this a lot with parents of children with health problems that may be addressed with food changes. Even if one parent is ready to make this a priority, the other one may not be on board and this makes for a rocky start. Unless the health issues are severe, they know it will take time and effort to address their child's ailment(s) and they simply don't have the energy. It's not our job to judge. We all have our limit to the amount of change or chaos we can handle at any point in time. It's a matter of self-preservation. I felt the same way about getting a dog and having a third child. I knew our family would benefit greatly from both, but I simply didn't have the stamina and knew it would easily send me right over the edge.

Sarah is another good example of being in denial. She has Hashimoto's (an autoimmune disease) with interstitial cystitis and is in pain. She is treating her condition with a variety of medications and surgeries, which aren't helping much. Sarah's mother knows that she is addicted to junk food, but she is at college and not ready to discuss the idea that changing her food could improve her symptoms.

What if you hit the tipping point for someone else you care about? Please understand that you cannot force someone to change their eating if they don't want to. It's like forcing a smoker to quit when they aren't ready, even if they have lung cancer. They must hit the tipping point all on their own. Talking about healthy eating incessantly to a husband who is recouping from triple bypass but lives on steak and fries is just going to send him running. Try using the tips and tools provided in this book to help them make small changes that build up over time. Do more and talk less. Eventually, they will start to feel better and begin to see the relationship between changes in their diet and decreases in their symptoms. It should start to gain momentum from there.

Something strange happens right after you hit your tipping point. **The universe may start speaking to you.** You will notice more and more stories of people going through a similar situation. It's like when your family is expecting a baby and, all of a sudden, everyone is pregnant around you! Maybe you tore your ACL and now you hear of three people who have recently had the surgery and it seems like countless news articles are all talking about torn ACLs. When I first tried a grain-free eating style, the author of *The Caveman Diet* happened to be a guest on my favorite radio program. Ironically, at that time, even my mother-in-law, who ate white bread and almost no veggies her entire life, explained that she was trying a grain-free diet to address some of her maladies. I can't explain it. It's like being in a Twilight Zone episode. All I can say is, if the universe speaks to you, just listen and say, "Thanks for the encouragement."

Everyone hits their own tipping point before deciding to make a change. Whether you are forced to make this change or you are inspired to proactively take control of your health, this change model will help guide you through the transition, step by step.

PERSONAL BITE

I used to think I was so healthy. Everyone who knew me said the same thing because I looked that way on the outside. Ironically, I even bragged that I was a "healthy" eater just because I didn't eat a ton of junk food anymore. But looks can be deceiving. Part of me was in denial and the other part of me had no idea how much better I could feel. Learning to live with a host of small health problems was just part of life, including these new waves of numbness and tingling in my left leg. But one night, as I laid in bed, the waves in my left leg didn't stop. My right leg started, then both arms and into my face (reminding me of the early signs of Bell's palsy I had years before). I knew I'd hit my tipping point and couldn't ignore this problem any longer. It was like a switch went off. I wasn't sure where I was headed, but I knew there was no going back.

BUSINESS BITE

Just as you can get comfortable with the current state of your diet and your health, businesses can also become complacent with the status quo. A company blindsided by their competition may reach a tipping point when they are inevitably forced into making a major change to catch up. Very successful companies incorporate constant change into their culture, so they always stay ahead of the curve.

Netflix is a great example of a company who hit their tipping point and embraced change every step of the way. Netflix started in 1997 as a company offering DVD rentals by mail. Not long after, they were the first to provide customers with a monthly DVD subscription service with unlimited rentals, no due dates, late fees, or shipping costs. Netflix continued to seek change and evolve, launching their internet streaming service. Their success completely caught TV networks off guard. In 2018, Netflix plans to spend $8 billion[10] producing their own original content. They now reach a global audience of around 118 million people[11] dominating the streaming video market.

BEFORE YOU BITE

What's changed for you? Have you hit your tipping point? Maybe you have always been health conscious but now want to change how you eat to be more environmentally conscious as well. Perhaps you are fed up with your own growing list of health challenges and have decided that enough is enough. No matter how you eat today, there is always room to improve how we eat and how we feel.

If you are reading this book, my guess is that if you haven't already reached your tipping point, you are probably very close, perhaps peeking over the edge. Take some time to reflect on this now. Your tipping point will act as your anchor and you will undoubtedly come back to it for inspiration at various points in your journey.

MY TIPPING POINT

Describe the moment you had enough and decided to change? Where you were and what happened? If it didn't happen yet, what would it look like?

_____

_____

_____

_____

_____

_____

_____

SAVOR IT: Once you are finished, take a step back and reflect on your tipping point. Do you have the feeling that "enough is enough" and something has to change? Do you have a current health problem or are you motivated by the idea that your health could be even better than it is now?

Envision Health

Create a Personal Health Vision

—

Assess "Stomach" for Change

—

Study Yourself

1

CHAPTER FOUR

1 Envision Health

The answer to the question, "Why change?" is not always as obvious as you think. You may be tempted to simply answer, "So I am free from illness," but that is only the tip of the iceberg. Why do you want to be free from illness? What does this allow you to do in your life that is so important? Digging down to reveal these answers helps you envision your health in a way that is truly compelling.

You may not realize it now but there are a whole host of benefits you will discover once you transform your health. You have no idea how sick you are until you are better! Perhaps you will sleep soundly for the first time and wake up energized in the mornings, you may get sick less often and get better faster, or improve your sex life! So many aspects of health are possible for you!

Before you select a specific diet or food plan, it's important to take a moment (yes, go slow to go fast) to assess your readiness or "stomach" for change and what types of foods your body responds to best. This is your first "language" class where you will begin to interpret some of the most basic messages your body tells you every day.

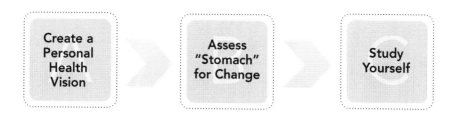

Create a Personal Health Vision

Health is a completely relative term. Each of us has a different vision or picture of what "perfect" health looks and feels like and why it's so important to achieve. Professional athletes may define health as having the strength and flexibility to achieve their sports goals. Another person may describe perfect health as the ability to participate in a local 5K, while others who struggle with illness may define health as simply making it through the day without pain. Earlier, we reflected on our own personal stories of how we arrived at this point in our lives and our health. Now, let's take some time to visualize exactly what health looks and feels like to you in the future.

PERSONAL BITE

My quest for answers produced a lot of anxiety, which made my symptoms worse. I went to multiple doctors and wellness practices over the course of three years and was grasping at straws, looking for a solution. I became obsessed with food, treatments, and my symptoms—it was all I could think and talk about. Books, online research, countless visits and wellness treatments later, I finally put the pieces together from a variety of sources. But changing my entire diet wasn't exactly the silver bullet I was hoping for. Like countless other patients, I was told to give up over 50% of the foods I was eating, given some supplements, and sent on my way. Good luck with that.

It quickly became clear "what not to eat," but exactly how to go about doing that left me a bit paralyzed. It felt like I was standing on the edge of a cliff and someone told me to get across to the other side, but there was no bridge in sight. **The reality is that the decision to change alone, without a clear vision and structured process to get there, is not enough to achieve success.**

I decided to take a step back and look at the big picture. What exactly was on the opposite side of the cliff anyway and was it really worth the effort? Following my own change management consulting advice, I started to create a clear and compelling vision. I dared myself to imagine my life with perfect health. I mapped out the symptoms I wanted to address, but more importantly, how I would feel and what I would do once they were gone. I started to imagine my life as an empty nester with my husband in the future, enjoying a trip to Italy, a casual game of tennis, strolling around farmer's markets, and stand-up paddling in the ocean. There was no time for sickness, pain, or naps of out necessity in this picture. When my vision was complete, something shifted in my mind and body, and it was for the better. It was then that I decided not only was I going to achieve my vision, but I would write a book about my journey and the structured process I used to get there.

BUSINESS BITE

Most change experts agree that businesses need a compelling vision for change and it must be communicated clearly to all employees. Everyone in the organization needs to understand why this change is needed now and how it could affect them if not addressed. Is the business lagging behind the competition? Perhaps an immediate response to strong customer feedback is necessary. Understanding the impetus for the change is key to getting everyone on board to support it.

As consultants, inevitably, we go into an organization to address one issue but find that our solution solves a whole host of other business problems. For example, a company may select a new technology solution to streamline business processes but, surprisingly, it may also provide some much needed customer service data to improve target marketing of new products. You, too, will find that when you set out to improve one set of symptoms, a whole host of other health problems are remarkably improved as well! A deep understanding of why change is necessary and a comprehensive vision of all that is possible in the future is key to success.

BEFORE YOU BITE

It's important to create an inspiring health vision that will keep you motivated throughout your transformation. Losing weight is often not a powerful enough incentive. Instead, identify the specific health improvement you would like to see. Take the time to acknowledge why your health is so important and all that is possible once you achieve it. You may dream of a special vacation with your family or simply the ability to walk your favorite trail with your dog every day. With strength, high energy, full mobility and the absence of pain, anything is possible.

Personal Vision Activity Visualization has long been a powerful tool for achieving your goals. The most effective vision captures not necessarily what you want to achieve but how you will feel once you obtain it. I have used the personal vision exercise successfully with employees facing massive organization changes as well as with individuals faced with the challenge of changing their diet to support a health problem.

To create your vision, ask yourself the following questions:

1. What are 2 things I would like to change about my health today?

Identifying your short-term goals helps identify and prioritize what is most important to you. Perhaps you want to address your frequent headaches, acid reflux, joint or muscle pain, bloating, eczema, acne, cold sore outbreaks, or chronic fatigue. Focusing on just a couple of high-impact areas is a great place to start.

2. What aspects of my health would I like to address in the long-term?

Think of your long-term goals like a holiday wish list. Maybe you want to achieve normal blood work results, repair your gut lining, strengthen your immune system, or prevent a family history of illness. Perhaps you just want solid, uninterrupted, deep sleep every night!

_____

_____

_____

3. Why change now?

Who and what is most important to you today? How does your health affect them or the current situation? Can you postpone the change, and if so, for how long?

_____

_____

_____

4. What will I do with "perfect" health in the future (3-5 years or more)?

It can be a bit scary to dare and think about all that is possible with amazing health. The sky is the limit with this question so dream big and small.

_____

_____

_____

SAVOR IT: Do you have a few symptoms that don't seem to add up? Consider a functional doctor or nutrition therapy practitioner to help you find the root cause of your health problem. Obtaining or ruling out a diagnosis such as leaky gut, Lyme disease, celiac disease, or adrenal fatigue can help make your health vision a reality sooner than later.

Now, create a visual depiction of your personal health vision. Take some time to make it your own. Add words, phrases, pictures, or anything else that represents your vision. Once completed, post it somewhere to keep you inspired and motivated throughout your journey.

Identify your personal motto below your vision. Your motto is a phrase that simply represents how you approach life. It doesn't have to be deep so don't think too hard about it. My personal motto is, "Go slow to go fast," as evidenced many times in my life and throughout this book!

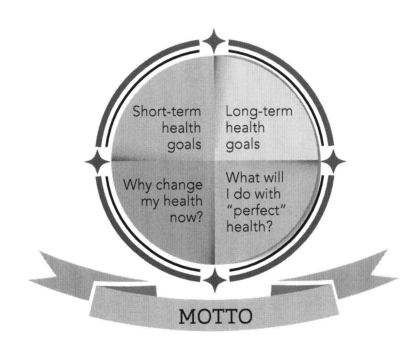

PERSONAL HEALTH VISION

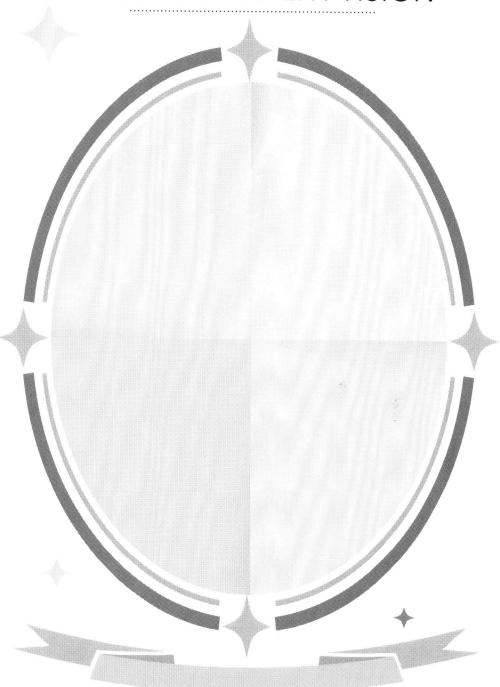

Assess Your "Stomach" for Change

Individuals and businesses all have their own threshold or "stomach" for change. It's important to recognize your level of change readiness early in the process so you can plan accordingly. The bigger the change, the more discomfort you may encounter. Many people faced with change say they have a physical reaction, such as a pit or twisting feeling in their gut. Consider how you felt when you signed your name with your opposite hand. Now, imagine visiting another country and driving on the opposite side of the road! How uncomfortable would that feel?

The routine of our lives brings us comfort, calmness, and control. When we disrupt that routine, it is natural to react with fear or discomfort. Change is often difficult, so unless the benefits outweigh the effort, many choose the status quo. Your change readiness may vary based on a few factors: the magnitude of the change (How big of a deal is it?), the sense of urgency (How quickly does it need to happen?) and the rewards to be gained (Are the health benefits worth the effort?). Be honest. How would you assess each of these factors as it relates to your own food and wellness goals? What else might impact your ability to make a change?

As you are faced with the idea of changing how you eat, try to acknowledge the feeling of discomfort and not judge it. Most people have a physical, emotional, or even violent reaction to the idea of giving up any kind of food such as dairy, processed foods, gluten, meat, or sugar. Don't worry. This feeling of anxiety can protect you from making too many rash decisions all the time! You may need a little time to "digest" the idea of eating differently. But whether you have decided to cut down a little, give up entire categories of food all together, or to simply add more fruits and veggies to your plate, it all requires some form of change. We will use your current readiness or "stomach" for change to develop a transition plan and pace of change that's right for you.

PERSONAL BITE

Honestly, I don't think I would have ever given up grains (later, just gluten) and dairy without having a health problem. I'm 100% Italian after all, which means that bread, pasta, and cheese practically run through my veins. In my family, we plan the next meal before we are finished eating the current one. After assessing my own readiness or "stomach" for change, well, let's just say I needed to practice what I had preached all these years. When the practicality of it all set in, it was clear that I was both physically addicted and emotionally connected to so many foods. Just the idea of giving them up was painful. I needed to make life-long changes to food habits that had developed since childhood in the hopes of improving my symptoms. While my head was convinced a food change was necessary for my health, my heart was holding on, sad to say goodbye to foods I loved.

It was hard not to jump ahead and get caught up in the emotions of it all. I thought about Christmas, the seven fishes dinner (Italian feast with a variety of fish and pasta dishes), and the smell of anisette from making pizzelles. These were a huge part of my Christmas season as a child and are now part of my own family's tradition. These were important food memories that included my mother, grandmother, and other family members who had passed away, so it was particularly hard to let them go.

Recognizing my own "stomach" for change was important because it helped me set the pace and approach for my food transition to ensure long-term results. For example, I took a few weeks to test out my new way of eating while letting some off-limit foods slip through the cracks just to build my confidence. The idea of never eating ice cream at the beach again for the rest of my life was a bit too much to handle. Even though all grains were off limits initially, I found that a gluten-free cookie during the holidays was exactly what my body and heart needed for long-term success.

BUSINESS BITE

Some companies are slower to change than others. But why? This has little to do with industry type, size, or location, but rather the company's readiness for change. We often assess this by using surveys and interviews to learn more about their experience with change (good and bad) as well as the culture of change within the leadership team and with employees.

Some companies make change an integral part of their culture and are far more adept at it. Others are bogged down by bureaucracy, resulting in slow-moving or no change at all. It may be difficult to take the same transformation program from a small, nimble, and "change ready" company and implement it in a large financial services corporation. Just as businesses align their pace of change with the company culture to optimize the benefits over the long-term, we need to match our food transition plan with our own "stomach" for change.

BEFORE YOU BITE

The first time I talk to a potential health coaching client, I go through a change readiness assessment process. I ask questions to confirm they are ready physically and emotionally to take on the challenge. While I do try and get a general sense of their food habits and the extent of their palette, this is less important than my client's willingness to change. I don't care if they eat doughnuts for breakfast, lunch, and dinner. What I care most about is their desire to make improvements to their food and health, no matter how small. This process also gives me a sense of how to plan their transition. The rate and speed of change varies dramatically from one person to the next.

Rachel is a good example of developing a short-term plan based on her current "stomach" for change. She was recently diagnosed with hypothyroidism and is taking medication while currently caring for her sick father. She knows her diet dramatically affects her symptoms but is not able to shop and cook at home right now. Being realistic about her situation, she makes only minor changes to her diet during the day but decides to temporarily subscribe to a meal prep delivery service that fits her dietary restrictions for dinner. She also keeps a few organic frozen meals on hand to help her in a pinch. When

Rachel is more "ready," she will begin shopping and cooking on a regular basis. This approach allows her to begin seeing some health benefits, which will incentivize her to continue making progress as her situation improves in the future.

Consider other change events going on in your life now. Did you recently lose a parent? Are you going through a divorce? Is your child having a hard time in school? There is never a good time to be sick or to get healthy, but you can move forward if you adjust your pace of change to accommodate your current situation. How ready are you to make a change today? What is your "stomach" for change on a scale of 1-10?

_____

_____

_____

_____

_____

SAVOR IT: Consider your eating habits and the diversity of your food palette today. Do you think the change will be easier or harder than you initially assessed? How might this impact how quickly you plan to transition to a new way of eating?

"Change is hard at first, messy in the middle, and gorgeous at the end." — *Robin Sharma*

Study Yourself

Before you identify a new eating strategy and wellness practices to support your health vision, you must first learn more about the foods that work best for you. Throughout this process, you will get to know your body better than any scientist, specialist, or expert out there. You will become hyper aware of how different foods interact with your physical and emotional state better than ever before. You will have a mindful connection to your body that is extremely powerful, and this will benefit you for the rest of your life. Equipped with this new superpower, you may find yourself diagnosing the reason for your mild headache, bloating, or new rash on your face. Your body is constantly communicating with you and you are simply a student of the language.

Think of understanding messages we receive from our body as interpreting an infant's cry. It may not be obvious at first, but after a lot of time and practice, you begin to understand exactly what your body's problem is and how to fix it. You may not like what your body is telling you and feel angry or deny the problem all together, but you can't "unknow" it, just like the smell of a dirty diaper.

Forget about the word "diet" and focus on the health problem you are trying to solve (big or small) and use that as the incentive to change how you eat. For example, giving up dairy doesn't feel nearly as hard if you are trying to reduce excess mucus in your nose and throat and prevent gas.

I love listening to other people's stories about their food sensitivities and "trigger" foods, even though they all sound exactly alike. All stories begin with a particular food they loved and ate all the time. The journey through discovery begins when they start to recognize possible symptoms and realize that this food may be a potential problem. The process of testing the theory and the food continues until a reluctant acknowledgment that indeed this "trigger food," does, in fact, wreak havoc on their bodies. After a bit more denial and testing, the story almost always ends with a triumphant tale of how giving up this food has changed their life and they have never felt better. It's like reality television—it's all the same, but I just can't get enough!

Vanessa is a great example of someone who suffered with heartburn and stomach aches. A New Year's resolution led her to try a detox and take several high allergen foods out of her diet. She then gradually added them back in one by one to test their impact on her symptoms. She was horrified to find that it was eggs, her favorite food, that were the culprit. After remaining in denial for a while, she continued to eat eggs and suffer with the consequences. Eventually, she couldn't "unknow" the problem anymore and finally stopped eating them and felt amazing.

Depending on how severe your reaction to the "trigger" food is, you may continue to test yourself until you have reached your tipping point all over again. Over 30% of people in the food transition survey told us that they couldn't resist cravings to restricted foods sometimes. Maybe you have celiac disease and that pigs in a blanket or chicken finger begs you to take a bite, and what happens? You tell yourself that one bite couldn't possibly hurt you, but, sure enough, you are sick as a dog, swearing off that food for life. This becomes a seesaw effect where you go back and forth until your mind, heart, and stomach are all in agreement. **The good news is that the sicker you feel after eating your "trigger" food, the easier it is to give it up.**

PERSONAL BITE

What sounded like a death sentence eventually turned into a blessing in disguise. I had no idea how certain foods were impacting my body. I was receiving messages every day and simply ignoring them. Something interesting happens when you begin to clean up your diet. You start to hear your body's language loud and clear. I realized after removing gluten and dairy from my diet that they were the culprit of so many problems including bloating, cysts on my face, and chronic congestion. Over time, I have learned to interpret almost everything my body tells me. Too much yeast and I cut back on sugar. Not enough sleep and my throat will get a mild pain, or I will feel a threatening cold sore in my nose. Too stressed and my nerve will spasm in my left leg. Even my body's odor will tell me when I've eaten too much meat. Too many vegetables and, actually, nothing happens. I just wanted to make sure you were paying attention! But this is exactly my point: we need to start paying attention to our bodies! You really will be amazed with what it has to say.

My own story of discovery with gluten:

I come from long line of Italian ladies with small bodies and big bellies. They always used to joke that it was "the bread" that did it. I guess they were right. One day, my grandmother lost her appetite, and after a year, her stomach literally exploded with undiagnosed stomach cancer. When my mother was in hospice, diagnosed with lung cancer (who knew smoking was bad back in the fifties?), I noticed something very interesting. She stopped eating her toast for only a couple days and her body looked completely different after such a short time. Her stomach was no longer bloated as I always knew it to be. It matched the rest of her small body for the first time, and she was in complete proportion.

Years later, I looked down at my own stomach after dinner, which included bread and butter. My stomach was so distended (again), I easily looked six months pregnant. I thought to myself, "It's got to be the bread." I have a small frame like my mom, but for years, I would wear clothes to fit my bloated belly so nobody could see just how disproportionate my body was and how uncomfortable I always felt. After I removed gluten from my diet, I couldn't believe the results. Just like my mom, I had finally uncovered the proportionate body I was supposed to have all along, only I didn't need cancer to help me find it.

BUSINESS BITE

Businesses undergoing a major change must also be honest and take a good, hard look at themselves to diagnose their problems. Maybe a top member of the executive team is acting counter to the culture and vision of the organization and it's the elephant in the room, but nobody wants to speak up. Perhaps your business model is successful today but has potential problems brewing in the future (think Blockbuster, circa 2002). Sometimes, there are problems in a company that nobody wants to admit, but once they are recognized and addressed, it can make all the difference in their future. Be honest about your health. Don't be afraid to admit when certain foods aren't working for you and need to be "fired."

BEFORE YOU BITE

How do you know what foods are right for you? So many recommendations and reports contradict each other. One week a food is good for you, and the next week, it's not. **The reality is that the same food can fuel one person and act as poison to another.** It's not whether a food is good or bad, but how it makes you feel that counts.

The best way to start learning about the foods you eat and the effects they have on your body is through a food and symptom diary. This is a great tool when you are just starting to identify how different foods make you feel. A food and symptom diary helps track what you eat, when you eat it, and how you feel afterwards. You track your physical and emotional responses to your meals immediately after eating, a few hours later, and later that night to see if you can find trends that map your symptoms with specific foods you consumed.

Don't ignore any reactions, track it all, even if you think it's not important. Make a note of ANY reactions, no matter how insignificant you think they may be (i.e. heartburn, diarrhea, rash, bloating, gas, breakout, cough, inflammation). I realized after going through this process with my own

FOOD & SYMPTOM DIARY

Date _____

Symptoms
(include specific time of symptoms)

Food/Drink

	Right after I ate it....	3 hours after I ate it...	Later that day/night...

BREAKFAST

LUNCH

DINNER

SNACKS

children that gluten made them downright angry and aggressive. After eating a good quality meal, you should feel great! If not, it's time to dissect your plate.

Use the food diary provided or use any method to document your food and related symptoms, like a food and symptom app on your phone, or make notes in a small book you keep with you. Eventually, this will become an intuitive process whereby you will see or feel something different in your body and immediately trace it back to your last meal and the possible food culprit.

SAVOR IT: Stop and reflect on your food diary. Do you see any patterns? Are you surprised by the results? Does this confirm some of your suspicions? What symptoms and patterns are still not clear and may require further testing?

No matter what your age, trust yourself and the information your body gives you. With continued awareness of what you are eating and how it makes you feel, you will soon become an expert in your own body's language.

Elimination Process If you have a host of symptoms that don't seem to map back to any one food, you may want to try an elimination process. An elimination is when you remove anywhere from one to all eight of the top allergens from your diet for at least four weeks. This includes eggs, milk, peanuts, tree nuts, soy, wheat, shellfish, and fish. I add corn to my client's list as I see a lot of sensitivities with it. One by one, introduce foods back onto your plate and test your reaction. If you are food sensitive, it won't take long for your symptoms to come out.

Consider your "stomach" for change when planning an elimination diet. Some people eliminate three or four foods at once while others do one at a time. If your diet contains primarily gluten, dairy and eggs, you may not want to eliminate all three at the same time or you will have nothing left to eat! It's way too much for some to handle while others want to get the process over with and will bear anything for a month just to get some answers.

"I suffered for years with a mystery illness. After I finally got diagnosed with celiac disease, I learned first-hand the power of diet, not only in my recovery to health, but in every aspect of day-to-day living. Before diagnosis, I didn't connect my health challenges to my on-going wellbeing. Since then, I've learned to listen to my body and have discovered that it talks to me all the time—sometimes loudly!"

— *Alice Bast, CEO of Beyond Celiac*

If you decide to eliminate gluten, make sure you do your research to thoroughly understand what it is and what foods contain it. Focus on foods that are naturally free of gluten, like vegetables, fruits, organic meats, beans, and nuts. There are some grains that contain gluten (like wheat, barley, and farro), so do some homework to learn how to read labels with ingredients containing hidden gluten. There are so many gluten-free resources available now with lots of information on products and trends in gluten-free eating, such as *Gluten-Free Living* and the *Celiac Disease Foundation*.

Try to focus on eating real foods and don't replace everything you eat today with a "gluten-free" version. Over-processed products are not good fuel for your body, gluten-free or not. **My suggestion is to pick only one or two things on your list of current foods that you simply cannot live without and transition to a gluten-free version of that.** All the grocery stores and even the dollar stores have picked up on the increase in demand and profit of gluten-free foods. So be careful and limit purchases to products with a limited number of ingredients that you can pronounce.

I met a woman who had been suffering with severe intestinal problems for years. I knew she ate almost all meals out at restaurants or take-out. When I asked her if she had tried a gluten-free diet, she responded, "I tried that, and it didn't work. I ate gluten-free pancakes, gluten-free bread, gluten-free cookies, gluten-free crackers, you name it. None of it helped." Gluten-free or not, processed food is not really food at all and won't make you magically better or thinner. In fact, it may make matters worse.

Take allergens out of your body that cause you trouble and replace them with nutritious real foods (perhaps some frozen berries or mixed nuts). You will be shocked at how amazing you begin to feel.

Is Cleaner Better? Many people suspecting a sensitivity (not allergy) tell me they don't want to remove certain foods because then their body won't be able to tolerate them anymore. Others say they don't want to know which foods are bad for them because ignorance is bliss. But is it? You will inevitably hone your skill to interpret the messages your body gives you about the food you eat. As more whole, nutritious foods become part of your diet, your body naturally rids itself of toxins, and these messages become even more clear. They start as a quiet whisper and, over time, they sound like a bullhorn, impossible to ignore. For example, I used to get the occasional headache or feel completely exhausted out of nowhere. But after learning to listen carefully to my body, I can usually tie a certain symptom back to something I ate and it all makes complete sense.

> *You will inevitably hone your skill to interpret the messages your body gives you about the food you eat.*

For example, a person with celiac, diagnosed at age thirty, may not have had any immediate reactions over the years when consuming gluten. However, once they take it out of their diet completely, they may start to see an immediate and strong response when "dosed" with foods that were even cross contaminated with gluten. Others may find that they are able to tolerate a small amount of certain "trigger" foods. Wouldn't you rather know now than ignore the symptoms for years until a bigger health problem arises? It's better to have the power and control to make a conscious decision and knowingly manage the consequences. It's like drinking contaminated water. It may or may not make you sick immediately, but wouldn't you want to know it was polluted before drinking it? Eventually, you will get addicted to feeling great and won't want the food you are sensitive to anyway.

After one person is diagnosed with a health problem or food sensitivity, it's easier to see how food may be impacting others in the family. I've seen a four-year-old test positive for celiac but her one-year-old sister test negative. Doctors told the parents they did not need to put the younger sister on a gluten-free diet. They were told to watch her carefully for similar gastrointestinal symptoms and have her tested every year for celiac for the rest of her life. Sure enough, within six months, and through her parent's careful observations, the one-year-old began showing similar symptoms and tested positive for celiac. Knowing what to look for made it so much easier to see the problem. Best of all, going through the change process was a breeze the second time around.

The goal is to teach everyone in your family at every age to be aware of changes in their body and how they may be reacting to certain foods. In my house, my son and I have a clear sensitivity to gluten and dairy, but my daughter did not show any signs. I showed her through my own journey what food reactions I experienced and what to look for. We don't talk about diets or "healthy" foods in our house. We focus on eating real food and how it makes us feel. As a result, when my daughter was ten years old, she came to me after eating ice cream and showed me her extremely distended belly. "Mom, I think I have a problem with dairy." I didn't have to say or do a thing.

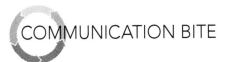

COMMUNICATION BITE

Remember that your support system is just as critical to your success as employees are to the companies they work for. Just as organizations must communicate a clear vision and reason for change to employees, you must do the same with your "tribe" of close family and friends about your vision of health.

Only 10% of people from the food transition survey "found it difficult sometimes to follow their dietary restrictions because they don't get help/support from family/friends (i.e. in the form of peer pressure, guilt, attitude)." Start by explaining your health problem and vision to your tribe.

Explain to them what you have discovered thus far in the process. Help them understand why this change is so important to you. They love you and can't help if they don't know what's going on.

Be prepared to specifically answer the question from your tribe, "What can I do?" Don't be afraid to ask for help. Would you help them if the situation was reversed? This is the awkward time to explain to your spouse that while you appreciate the thoughtful gesture of picking up your favorite cheesesteak, that it's not helping you achieve your health goals. Perhaps he could see if your favorite pizza place has a gluten-free crust or special salad? Help your tribe help you.

If you notice that someone is reacting negatively or perhaps even judgmental of your new eating strategy, trust me, it has nothing to do with you. **They are projecting fears of their own health and eating habits onto you.** This is not your battle to fight. We found in the food transition survey that almost 50% said they have not told someone about their diet restrictions for fear of being judged. My suggestion is to just lead by example and demonstrate how eating a certain way is a small price to pay for eliminating all your health problems and feeling amazing!

The first bite to health is arguably the most important step of all. Understanding why you want to change your eating habits and creating a vision for your future health is the first secret. By recognizing your willingness or "stomach" for change, you can plan an approach and pace of change that's just right for you. Now that you are armed with the knowledge of what foods work best for your body, you are poised to identify the best eating and wellness plan to achieve your health vision.

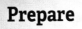

Prepare

Pinpoint Food/
Wellness Plan
—
Win Quick
—
Team Up

2

CHAPTER FIVE

2 Prepare

Now that you have defined exactly what health is and how it will feel once you have it, it's time to determine the best plan of attack for how to achieve it! In this chapter, you will identify an eating strategy or "food plan" that is aligned with the foods that work best with your body. You will also identify some specific wellness practices to combat your health concerns and/or help prevent health problems in the future. As with a business transformation, you will find ways to "win quick" by identifying several high impact actions to build confidence and create some momentum for change. Finally, you will begin to understand the power of teaming-up with others to create accountability and establish a support system to lift you up and support you along the journey.

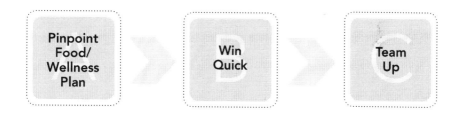

Pinpoint Your Food and Wellness Plan

There are many different approaches to help you achieve your health vision. Food is an integral part of your journey and selecting a food plan that matches your "stomach" for change is a great place to start. There are also a variety of wellness practices that can make a huge impact on your health goals. Let's review how to conduct some fundamental research to find the approach that works best for you.

Pinpoint a Food Plan   There are almost 73,000 health-related books, over 100 diet theories, countless reputable websites, and plenty of new documentaries outlining a variety of eating strategies that you can choose from. It may be easier to narrow down the list if you focus on a specific health goal or problem you want to solve or prevent in the future. For example, if you have diabetes or a heart condition, you can easily search for programs and resources targeted specifically for those issues.

If you have a specific health issue, consult with doctors, coaches, and other healing professionals for their suggestions. Ask everyone you feel comfortable with if they have any experience with your specific health problem(s) or goal(s) and find out what has or has not worked for them. You may be surprised by who is the most helpful. It could be your child's teacher, a co-worker, cousin, or neighbor who has the best experience and advice.

Review online bookstores and search using keywords that describe your health problem or interest area (i.e. inflammation, arthritis, grain-free, vegan). Watch food documentaries or wander around your local bookstore, paging through a variety of resources in the health section. Try to maintain perspective when doing your research and not become overwhelmed. Obtain enough information to motivate you without becoming paralyzed. Once you have a chance to review a variety of options, you will find a food plan that resonates with you and your "stomach" for change. You may also have a food plan in mind already or want to re-commit to one you used with success in the past. It doesn't have to be the perfect plan. Just pick one you feel will kickstart your progress. Keep in mind that the food plan you select may also change over time as trial, error, and adjustment will give you the best results.

Customize a Food Plan   You may find comfort and success in choosing one specific eating strategy and following it exactly as it is written, with no exceptions. But you may also want to custom design your own food plan.

This means that you pull different pieces out of different eating plans to create a customized solution. It's your life, your body and your health, so do what works best for you.

If you have a health problem, you may need to follow your food plan strictly at first to get your symptoms until control. In other cases, the 80% solution may also be effective. This business term refers to the strategy of investing only enough effort to complete 80% of your objective. I adjusted and applied this theory to my food plan by initially telling myself that I only had to follow the plan 80% of the time. Just the idea of telling myself I didn't have to eat grain, gluten, or dairy-free all the time took the pressure off. As soon as someone tells me I can't have something, suddenly it's all I want.

The 80% solution allowed me to look at a piece of bread and know I had a choice. I knew I would face the consequences of eating it, so I might ask, "Is it worth it?" Perhaps a piece of crusty Italian bread from South Philly would tempt me, but the freedom of choice gave me the control to decide for myself. Most times, I chose to say, "No, thanks," but if I did decide to eat it, I didn't need to eat the entire bread basket because the choice was mine. If I felt bloated, sick, or broke out on my face for two weeks, I owned it. Eventually, it just wasn't worth it anymore and I stopped eating gluten all together.

If you have a serious food allergy, this theory does not apply. It's like a doctor saying your appendectomy surgery was a success because he was able to take 80% of your appendix out. It's all or nothing in that case.

We used the 80% solution approach quite a bit on consulting projects. I led a project to create an entire new operational model (design of new call center, new organization structure, new technology, and shift in organization culture). With so much on our plate, we could have spent three years or more just designing everything in perfect detail before ever implementing a thing! The 80% solution helped us stay focused on key components of the design but not stress over small details. Occasionally, there was no room for error (i.e. determining headcount in the new organization structure), but overall, we stayed focus on the 80% solution, which allowed us to kick-start our progress and tweak it along the way.

Your food plan helps define what "healthy eating" means to you. The strategy, "I'm trying to eat healthier," is far too generic. People use this phrase all the time and it's confusing. While everyone can agree that candy and junk food is not good for you, the definition of "healthy eating" varies depending on your perspective. For example, "healthy" to one person might be a salad with grilled steak (low carb), while to someone else, it's vegetables and rice with beans (higher carb but vegan). A person striving to make a few small changes to their health might choose a small cheeseburger and salad with ranch dressing instead of a double burger with bacon and a side of fries. The next person might prefer a veggie burger with vegan cheese on a gluten-free roll, whereas someone else would never eat vegan cheese or a gluten-free roll because it's too processed! We need to remember that we are all different. Our unique food plan helps to clarify this. Maybe the old line "What's your sign?" should be replaced with "What's your food plan?"

It drives me crazy when people refer to some foods as a "special treat." My view is that we should adopt a food plan that makes us feel amazing and include some foods we don't normally eat in the plan itself. For example, I occasionally bake gluten-free cookies for my family. It's not a "treat" for following our food plan. It IS our food plan. If this food is included in our plan, then we don't give it any power and we certainly don't feel bad about eating it. Clearly, guilt has no home here.

While I may not agree with the government food pyramid, one of things I love about it is that it has a small space allocated for all the foods you're not supposed to eat too much of (i.e. fried foods, candy, etc.) at the top of the pyramid. Now, I don't believe that most people save this category for only once or twice a week as suggested, but what I love is that at least the graphic includes these foods and recognizes that sometimes we're going to eat them. When choosing a food plan, don't forget to allocate something into that space. Just don't call it a "treat" or I'll have to take you out for a walk.

Create a Wellness Plan It's your job to manage a blend of food and wellness practices that will bring you the most success. The treatments that you select will vary based on your current health status and goals. Talk to people you know to gather treatment suggestions and providers. You may decide to mix and match suggestions from multiple healing sources. For example, you may take supplements prescribed by your doctor or wellness practice, receive chiropractic care to alleviate any pain, use a meditation app on your phone for stress, and use essential oils to address anxiety at home.

Close to 40% of adults claim to use some type of alternative medicine.[12]

Some therapies are new and others date back thousands of years. Alternative therapies are gaining popularity for those who seek a different or complimentary solution to traditional pharmaceutical drugs.

A few wellness practices and treatments:

Acupuncture/Acupressure	Lymphatic Drainage
Aromatherapy/Essential Oils	Healing Massage
Ayurvedic Medicine	Mindfulness/Meditation
Biological Medicine	Neti Pot/Nasal Irrigation
Cannabidiol (CBD) Oil	Neuro/Bio-feedback
Chiropractic Care	Nutrition Therapy Practitioner
Colon Hydrotherapy	Reflexology
Energy Therapy	Reiki
Functional Medicine	Relaxation Techniques
Herbal and Chinese Medicines	Salt, Heat, and Light Saunas
Homeopathy	Supplements
IV Nutrient Treatments	Variety of Yoga Practices

Your sense of urgency and "stomach" for change will drive your wellness plan. If you have a condition or set of symptoms you want to get under control, you may take advantage of more aggressive wellness practices than someone proactively trying to stay ahead of their health. Don't wait until you have a problem to find alternative therapies. Research your local area to see what's available if and when you are ready to give it a try.

A relationship detox is also helpful to support your wellness and overall vision. Be honest about the people you surround yourself with to determine their role in your health. Are certain people in your life high-drama and do they give you anxiety? Perhaps their role in your life needs to take a backseat for a while. How would others describe your friendship and role in their lives? Reflect on how good of a friend you are to others and re-focus your time where it is most important.

PERSONAL BITE

My food plan was aimed at strengthening my nervous and immune systems and re-building my gut flora. I eliminated most processed foods completely and added a variety of fresh and fermented foods and drinks, rich in probiotics (i.e. sauerkraut, kombucha tea), into my diet. I used several treatments to detox the high metal levels in my body. I had multiple IV infusions, drank a metal detox supplement, and took several probiotics to heal my gut. I also used colon hydrotherapy and saunas to support elimination of toxins from my body. Meditation in some form became a daily practice whether it was 5-10 minutes using an app on my phone and/or a 20-minute guided meditation to ease me into sleep at night. Eventually, everything started to slow down, including my symptoms.

As I began to incorporate a variety of wellness treatments into my routine, I noticed that my trips to the local pharmacist had all but stopped. While the cost of alternative therapies was not covered by insurance, I was surely saving on doctor's bills and prescriptions!

BUSINESS BITE

Just as we have a variety of eating and wellness practices to help us achieve our vision, businesses also have a variety of strategies, structures, and technology solutions available to them to help make their vision a reality. Similarly, their sense of urgency for change and current culture are key factors when selecting the best plan of action. They may look to change their pricing strategy, incentive structure, or completely redesign the overall customer experience.

"Design thinking" uses the "go slow to go fast" mentality as they take the time needed to clearly define the problem the business is trying to solve before developing a solution to fix it. The question is not, "How do we sell more products to increase revenue?" but, "How do we describe our target customers and what is important to them? What kind of customer experience do they value and expect?" Asking and answering these deeper questions helps architect a comprehensive and more effective solution.

For example, banks that did not look to the future soon enough are losing customers to more creative payment solutions such as Venmo and Square. These apps incorporate a social experience into their products, which young customers of today value. Giving a facelift to their website or creating their own version of the payment system may help them in the short-term, but banks must look ahead to new technology and service solutions that give customers what they really want in the future.

BEFORE YOU BITE

Use the tips provided in this chapter to identify a food plan that will work best for your body, "stomach" for change, and vision. For example, if you are borderline hypoglycemic and need to eat frequent meals throughout the day, using the intermittent fasting method may not be your first choice. In the next chapter, we will review your current eating habits and compare them to those outlined in your new food plan. Then, we will outline a gradual transition to help you make the change.

Explore a variety of alternative or complimentary therapies to support your vision. Remember that food is the foundation, but there are so many other practices to improve your health. Discuss options with your doctor and use trial and error to determine which treatments give you the best results.

MY FOOD/WELLNESS PLAN

Summary of Food Plan: Identify one specific food plan or customize your own. Note the foods you plan to eat more of, less of, or eliminate all together.

_____

_____

_____

_____

_____

Summary of Wellness Plan: What types of wellness practices and treatments are you planning?

_____

_____

_____

_____

_____

_____

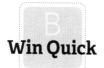

Win Quick

Using small successes to propel you forward helps create a momentum for bigger change. This is a good strategy for individuals taking on a new health vision and for businesses embarking on a transformation. You are more likely to act when you have just a few tasks to focus on at a time. You know the phrase, "How do you eat an elephant? ...One bite at a time." Identifying just a few small food and wellness changes each day or week is a great way to jumpstart your progress. This will give you a sense of pride and confidence in your ability to achieve your overall health vision. Take time as you go to recognize your accomplishments along the way and indulge yourself! Consider getting a spa pedicure or treat yourself to a new pair of jeans. Perhaps you could leave work a little early and take a walk at a nearby park or simply curl up on a rainy day and grab a quick nap.

One "win quick" example: John has heart disease and needs to clean up the processed foods in his diet. He does not have much of a "stomach" for change at all, but his wife decides to help him start with baby steps. The first goal is to switch from white bread to wheat bread. This may not seem like much but it's a big deal for John and he goes along. The second goal is to switch in a new breakfast of oatmeal with honey, nuts, and fruit instead of his daily routine of bacon and eggs. By constantly setting small goals each week, John establishes a new habit where little "change bites" become part of his everyday routine.

Clean out the kitchen. I am not a big fan of throwing everything out of your pantry and fridge that is not in your food plan on day one (unless, of course, you have a major allergy or health problem). Some "change ready" people find it helpful to wake up one morning and see no evidence of the way they used to eat. For the rest of us, I suggest a little straightening up. You get rid of a few major items but phase out the remaining foods in your kitchen over time. If you eliminate everything too quickly in the beginning, you might go food crazy when you step out into the real world of parties and restaurants. Think of straightening up the house before a few friends come over for dinner. No need to scrub every room. Clean up just enough to make a difference. It will be that much easier once you are ready for a full house cleaning.

PERSONAL BITE

When faced with the idea of cleaning out our basement, my husband and I have two different approaches. He is waiting for the perfect day when he can set out the dumpster bag and clean out the entire basement in one day. My strategy is to stop waiting and fill up one small contractor bag each weekend. Of course, we may end up with more than one bag if we get on a roll (which, of course, we will).

When I was faced with fundamentally changing everything I knew about my food habits, using the "win quick" strategy helped me break it down into manageable pieces. I quickly identified just a few quick meals I could keep on hand that would work within my new dietary restrictions. A batch of my new favorite detox soup with chicken, cannellini beans, and my favorite veggies was always in the fridge or freezer. Salad with all my favorite toppings, including avocado, sunflower seeds, lentils, pre-packaged grilled chicken strips, and beets, was ready to go for lunch or a snack. Mini egg frittatas became a staple in the house and I mixed up the ingredients each week. Having just a few meals and foods I could eat over the next few weeks gave me the confidence needed to reset my entire eating strategy.

BUSINESS BITE

When embarking on a large-scale change management initiative, we often incorporate the concept of "winning quick" early in the plan. In fact, a dedicated part of the project team is often allocated to achieving short-term improvements in the company in support of long-term goals. Realizing a few benefits early in the change process proves to employees that you are serious and committed to making positive improvements as quickly as possible. This also helps maintain a culture of constant change in the company.

I once led a dedicated "win quick" team for an insurance company as part of an overall transformation initiative. We were creating a new operational model and shifting to a results-oriented mindset as part of the new culture. Our project reviewed claims to identify and collect money owed but never collected. We tested a new process and brainstormed ideas for how to improve the customer service experience. We visually charted the results, including the total amount of money we collected. This was a fraction of the future savings, but it created some momentum and supported the long-term vision and new collaborative culture in the future.

BEFORE YOU BITE

You, too, can "win quick" by identifying and making a few changes immediately to set the stage for continuous change in your eating habits. Apply the basement cleanout scenario to guide your strategy. If your sense of urgency is high then, by all means, get the dumpster out and dive full force into your new food plan! If not, you may want to make a few changes to implement your plan gradually. Either way, taking the first step is the hardest so I suggest mastering one or two goals each day or week to get you started and create some positive momentum.

For example, try a few different non-dairy milks or switch to a new brand of your favorite oatmeal with less sugar. Find a new restaurant that caters to a variety of food intolerances. Consider a new style of food you wouldn't typically eat, such as Thai food. Consistently making a few small changes creates a new culture in your home and life where change is constant and expected. Think of culture as "how things are done around here." Get started today by writing down just a few things you can do tomorrow to build momentum for change in the future, and don't move on to new goals until these are accomplished.

WIN QUICK

What are a few small changes you can implement tomorrow to set the stage for continuous change?

Action	**Result**

Week 1:

Week 2:

Week 3:

Week 4:

Team Up

It's important that you team up with a variety of people who understand what you are going through and can help keep you accountable. Try to find special health interest groups on social media or find other Q&A or discussion groups online to ask questions and gain advice from others who truly understand. Only someone going through the same transition process can sympathize. It doesn't matter if you are managing a severe health problem, trying to prevent illness in the future, demonstrating animal rights, or supporting the environment. No matter what your goals are, we all need to connect to support and encourage each other!

Surround yourself with supportive people who really "get it."

PERSONAL BITE

Early in my food and wellness transition, I was at a school activity for my son and noticed that another mother had also declined the cookies and pretzels and mentioned she was gluten-free. We started talking and it turns out she had similar health issues and was also going through a metal detox while uncovering some food sensitivities along the way. Every time I saw her, we huddled together and talked about how we each felt and where we were in the process. We gave each other emotional support and practical tips such as recipes or new healing methods. She really understood what I was going through and that helped me a tremendous amount.

During this time, I found a Facebook page geared towards individuals striving to strengthen their nervous system and also joined several other discussion boards on the topics of eating grain and gluten-free. Eventually, I met more and more people with a variety of illnesses that used food as a primary healing method. So many random people in my life and community were going through a similar food and health transformation. Through this process, I found myself often using a favorite line from a fellow executive coach, "How can I help YOU?" Her theory about business networking was that if you focus on how to help others first, you will, in turn, benefit many times over. This was exactly the case when it came to "teaming up" with others on a similar health journey. The more I tried to help others, the more I gained in return.

BUSINESS BITE

Businesses recognize the value of teaming up with others for support. Many organizations embarking upon a major change in their business look to consultants to guide and support them in the process. Businesses may also team up by joining an industry association to share best practices with others. In *Cracking the Code of Change*, Beer and Nohria agree that "consultants can provide specialized knowledge and technical skills that the company doesn't have, particularly in the early stages of organizational change".[13]

Consulting is about teamwork, trust, and building relationships. I coached executives behind the scenes on how to lead their change initiatives, and we worked together to gain strong support from employees. I facilitated design sessions in a way that the client always felt ownership for the results. My industry expertise in change management coupled with their deep business knowledge was a powerful combination. Businesses can't be expected to know it all, and neither can you.

BEFORE YOU BITE

How will you "team up" with others you trust to help you on your journey to health? Who do you think will be particularly supportive? Which discussion groups can you find online? Are there social media sites that support your food and wellness plan (i.e. Instagram or Facebook)? Are there any local support groups or communities organized around your health goals or condition?

Take some time to document from who and how you can get the support you need to implement your new food and wellness plan right away. Consider working with a local health coach to support your transition and keep you accountable. If it's not in the budget now, maybe you could swap services with someone else. Early in my health coaching career, I swapped services with a personal trainer and it was a win-win for both of us!

How and with who will you team up with to support your health journey?

_____

_____

_____

COMMUNICATION BITE

The need for support along this bumpy ride of change cannot be stressed enough. You may have shared your initial diagnosis, condition, or allergy with your tribe early on, but keep them informed so they can keep supporting you. Be sensitive to the amount of minute details you share. For example, you may want to spare the specifics of each food sensitivity and reaction you experience. Sharing which treatment, supplement, or findings from your last colon hydrotherapy may be a bit too much information for most. I remember seeing the glazed looks in my friend's eyes as I went on and on about a new treatment therapy or food sensitivity. You can also risk sounding like a crazy person to someone who has no experience in following a new food plan or navigating a difficult health journey. Test your audience and proceed with care.

Tell your tribe how to help you. They may have no interest in following your food plan themselves and they may not have (or acknowledge) any of their own health problems, but it doesn't mean they don't care about yours. Let them know how to help you, even if it's just lending a sympathetic ear when you need to vent. Swap "I'm okay" with "This is hard and I'm struggling" and I guarantee those who care about you will provide you with the encouragement you need. Expect to feel a bit lonely early in your food change but resist the temptation to hibernate. Force yourself to meet up with a member of your tribe for coffee or a quick lunch—somewhere with plenty of food options. Take some time to listen to your friend's problems instead of focusing on your own for a while. Your buddy may have a funny story about his toddler or perhaps a friend could bend your ear to discuss a problem at work. Helping someone else is a great distraction and will inevitably help you, too.

The second bite to health is all about proper planning and communication early in the change process. Taking the time to create a food and wellness plan that is customized to your individual needs and goals will increase your chances for success down the line. Implementing a few changes to "win quick" early in the planning process will give you a sense of accomplishment. Teaming up with others provides the added support and motivation you need to persevere.

Commit

Identify Personal
Best Foods
—
Develop
Transition Plan
—
Simplify the
Process

3

CHAPTER SIX

3 Commit

"The rubber hits the road," as they say, in the third bite to health! In order to commit to this new way of eating, we begin to synchronize the way you eat today with the food plan you selected for the future. A customized transition plan will show respect to the food you love today and use it as a bridge to introduce additional nutritious, delicious foods onto your plate. I will also show you how to sharpen your own change consulting skills by streamlining the process of shopping and cooking to save time and money.

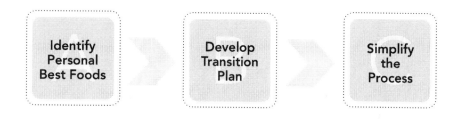

Identify Personal Best Foods

Now that you have identified a new food plan, you probably think we are ready to jump in and get started. But not so fast. Let's start by identifying your personal best foods. These are any whole foods (i.e. fruits, vegetables, grains, nuts, peas, beans) that you currently eat and enjoy. I find that even the pickiest eaters have a few "odd" whole foods that they enjoy. One client won't eat anything but junk, but he also loves Brussel sprouts. Another one eats only pasta, but will devour filet mignon and a bowl of pickles.

This strategy helps us to focus on the foods you CAN have instead focusing on the foods you CAN'T have.

PERSONAL BITE

While the idea of giving up certain foods was a little easier now that I understood how they negatively impacted me, I still couldn't help feeling a bit depressed about it all. I imagined myself pathetically eating a bowl of raw carrots or broccoli by myself while everyone around me was laughing and eating tons of amazing food. So, after a while, I decided to shift my thinking and make a list (okay, it was a spreadsheet, always a consultant) of all the whole foods I could eat. I was surprised at how long the list was! How did I forget about all those amazing foods?

I started keeping lists of all the fruits, vegetables, beans, and nuts I liked and used them as shopping lists. I began to incorporate them into all the recipes I was using while eliminating the other foods. Eventually, I used the variety of fresh produce in the store to guide my shopping and forgot the list all together. My energy and attention were now focused on all the new foods I could have and how I could creatively incorporate them into my meals. This positive shift made a huge difference in my own transition and became an important part of my personal best food strategy as a health coach in the future.

BUSINESS BITE

Organizations would never begin implementing a new strategic vision on day one without truly understanding their current business first. In fact, many companies assess their strengths or "core competencies" and use that as a foundation for their transition plan. These core competencies should not inhibit a company's ability to develop a creative and fundamentally different vision for the future, but it is quite helpful when determining an appropriate transition strategy. When planning for change, it just makes sense to start with what you are good at and expand from there. This is the exact model we will use for your food transition.

Let's use Amazon as an example. One of Amazon's core competencies is order fulfillment. You probably have a package at your front door right now. They have homed in on this customer-driven process with great success. Now, look at the recent purchase of Whole Foods by Amazon. In contemplating the merger, it makes sense for Amazon to take advantage of their existing customer service model and apply it to delivering Whole Foods groceries. By lowering prices on certain target foods, they are also trying to appeal to an even broader audience beyond their new combined customer base.

So, how can we apply all of this to your food plan? Just because you don't like vegetables doesn't mean that a vegan food plan is a bad idea. What it does mean is that you need to identify the only two vegetables you do eat and begin to expand into a transition plan from there instead of going 100% vegan tomorrow.

BEFORE YOU BITE

When identifying your own personal best foods, I want you to identify the foods that feel good to you physically and mentally. **Don't checkmark the foods you think you should eat just because you think they are good for you.** If kale disgusts you, then don't include it. Over time, with the addition of other green vegetables, you may eventually grow to love kale, but for now, keep it off the list.

It reminds me of a time I was reviewing a personal best list with a client who has a choking reaction to foods that she is sensitive or allergic to. When reviewing the list together, she told me, "I should be eating peppers because I'm not actually allergic and they are healthy for me. But they make me nervous and I think that I might choke on them." This food was clearly not good for her emotionally so there was no need to mark it as a personal best food. In fact, it made me want to create a personal worst list after that meeting.

PERSONAL BEST FOODS

Mark "2" next to the foods you like today and "1" next to the foods that you would try in the future. Leave the rest blank for now.

Vegetables

__ Acorn/Winter Squash

__ Artichoke

__ Asparagus

__ Avocado

__ Beet (red, yellow, orange)

__ Bell Peppers (red, green, yellow, orange)

__ Broccoli

__ Broccolini/Broccoli Rabe

__ Brussels Sprouts

__ Butternut Squash

__ Cabbage

__ Carrot

__ Cauliflower

__ Celery

__ Corn/Baby Corn

__ Cucumber

__ Edamame (soybeans)

__ Eggplant

__ Fennel

__ Green Beans

__ Greens - Bok Choy

__ Greens - Collard

__ Greens - Escarole

__ Greens - Kale (cooked)

__ Greens - Spinach (cooked)

__ Greens - Swiss Chard

__ Mushrooms _____

__ Olives

__ Parsnip

__ Peas

__ Potato (white, red, blue)

__ Radish

__ Rutabaga

__ Spaghetti Squash

__ Sugar Snap/Snow Peas

__ Sun-dried Tomato

__ Sweet Potato/Yam

__ Tomato

__ Turnip

__ Water Chestnuts

__ Yellow Squash

__ Zucchini (green squash)

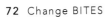

Fruit

— Apple
— Apricot
— Banana
— Blackberry
— Blueberry
— Cantaloupe
— Cherry
— Clementine/Tangerine
— Cranberry
— Dates

— Figs
— Grapefruit
— Grapes
— Honeydew
— Kiwi
— Lemon
— Lime
— Mango
— Nectarine
— Orange

— Peach
— Pear
— Pineapple
— Plum
— Pomegranate
— Pumpkin
— Raspberry
— Strawberry
— Watermelon

Nuts & Seeds

— Almonds
— Cashews
— Chia Seeds
— Coconut

— Flax Seeds
— Peanuts
— Pecans
— Pistachios

— Pumpkin Seeds
— Sesame Seeds
— Sunflower Seeds
— Walnuts

Beans & Peas

— Adzuki Beans
— Baked Beans
— Black Beans
— Black-eyed Peas
— Cannellini Beans
— Garbanzo Beans (Chickpeas)

— Kidney Beans
— Lentils
— Lima Beans
— Navy Beans
— Pinto Beans
— Split Peas

Grains

— Amaranth

— Barley

— Buckwheat

— Bulgur Wheat

— Millet

— Oatmeal

— Pasta (GF/Wheat)

— Quinoa

— Teff

— Rice (Brown, White, Wild)

Salad Greens

— Arugula

— Butter/Leaf Lettuce

— Escarole

— Iceberg Lettuce

— Kale (Salad)

— Microgreens

— Mixed Greens

— Romaine Lettuce

— Spinach (Salad)

— Watercress

Protein

— Beef: _____

— Chicken: _____

— Pork: _____

— Turkey: _____

— Fish: _____

— Tofu

— Tempeh

— Egg

Flavor

— Garlic

— Ginger root

— Hot Peppers

— Leek

— Onion (Sweet, Vidalia, Purple)

— Scallion

— Shallot

— Tumeric

SAVOR IT: Stop and reflect on your initial list of personal best foods. Are you surprised by the results? Is the list larger or smaller than you thought it would be? What foods did you forget that you liked because you haven't eaten them in a while?

Even my pickiest clients are often surprised by how many whole foods are included. If your list of whole foods is small, even simply two to three, don't worry! It doesn't matter where you start from, it matters that you move forward. Small change is better than no change at all.

Summarize your personal best food list in one page to make food shopping easier. Keep your list somewhere in sight or post it on your fridge to remind you of all the nutritious foods you enjoy eating and take the focus away from all the foods you can't or shouldn't eat. But keep the entire list on-hand so you keep the big picture in mind, outlining all of the possible food choices that await.

Develop a Transition Plan

Your "stomach" for change will guide the pace of your transition plan. Set realistic goals that factor in your resistance level and build confidence. A few gradual changes can make a big difference to your health over time. Plan the pace of change that's right for you.

Perhaps you have a host of symptoms that must be addressed immediately, or maybe you read about a new diet or detox and can't wait to get started. That's awesome! You can follow the guidelines for a successful transition no matter how fast or slow you plan to take it.

Here are a few client examples of using a gradual transition planning process:

Evan decides he wants to eat less red meat and more vegetables to reduce his cholesterol. He is resistant to changes in his diet. He puts ground turkey on his personal best list. He begins a slow transition to a variety of dishes made with ground turkey, such as a turkey burger, turkey meatloaf or meatballs, turkey tacos with veggies, ground turkey/vegetable tomato sauce, etc. He later tries turkey chili, adding some vegetables and beans. As a result, Evan eventually adds more veggies and beans to all his dishes.

Sean has been suffering with juvenile arthritis, so his mom decides to try introducing more whole foods into his diet to reduce inflammation. He is a very picky eater and highly resistant to change. His diet is very limited and includes pizza, mac n' cheese and chicken fingers. She sets very small goals that he can try right away. She experiments with adding a diced veggie or two (on his personal best list) to his pizza, and adding some chopped, cooked cauliflower to his mac n' cheese. Sean's mom begins making chicken fingers from scratch and later switches to grilled chicken strips dipped in BBQ sauce. Over time, she upgrades his mac n' cheese to pasta with chopped broccoli in olive oil with a sprinkle of parmesan cheese.

Mia gets severe stomach pains when she eats gluten, so she is transitioning to a gluten-free diet. She likes to eat pasta with butter, so she transitions to a brown rice pasta first and later begins adding a few veggies from her personal best List. She adds some chopped zucchini and cooked carrots and later some spinach and mushrooms into the dish. Over time, the pasta looks like a gourmet meal and Mia devours it!

When beginning to add vegetables to a dish (for both children and adults), it helps to start with a small amount and cut it into smaller pieces. For example, it you don't love mushrooms but are willing to try them, you shouldn't put a giant portobello in your pasta dish. Try chopping up some white button mushrooms to get used to the flavor and texture first. For some extremely resistant to change, simply adding some parsley to get used to seeing a green color in their pasta is progress. Smoothie drinks or bowls are another way to gradually introduce some greens, nuts, and seeds into your food. Start with a small handful of spinach (even a few leaves for the pickiest of eaters) and move forward from there.

Once you have settled into a new routine, keep only the food you want to eat in the house, including a few sweets. I remember, years ago, finding my young son upstairs, eating a bag of chocolate cream cookies and I thought, "WHAT are you doing?" Then I realized that if I bought it, they are going to eat it. Crazy concept, huh? I keep homemade banana muffins with a few mini chocolate chips or some dark chocolate in the house so nobody feels deprived. The reality is that I don't miss certain foods anymore because I'm not surrounded by them every day. More importantly, I'm addicted to how I feel without them. Until your kids can drive, you are the one who decides what food comes into the house. If you or someone in your family is a picky eater, use the transition plan to make improvements over time. Bottom line: do more and talk less. I see way better results when I don't talk too much about our food. I just buy and cook what I think we should all eat using the transition plan as a guide.

Identify ways to substitute ingredients in your family recipe so you don't have to lose the traditions. My sister perfected gluten-free pizzelles that taste better than the original, and nobody even noticed when we substituted gluten-free capellini into the seven fishes dinner! I now make the most incredible gluten-free, dairy-free lasagna with almond cheese, you would never know the difference!

Focus on the activity, not the food. Remember that the best part about making cookies with your mother or grandmother was the time you spent together. If you are transitioning to a vegan diet, don't be sad about the turkey at Thanksgiving. Focus on the tradition at the dinner table when you go around the table and each person states what they are thankful for. You can't buy that tradition, and you can't eat it either.

PERSONAL BITE

Because my symptoms were out of control, I had no choice but to make some dramatic changes immediately. I used my personal best foods as a starting point and then quickly began transitioning to a full set of meals aligned with my new dietary restrictions. I was surprised by all the wonderful food options available to me! There were plenty of food blogs and Instagram sites to provide me with inspiration. I made some adjustments to the food I love today, and the transition really started to take off! I made fish and chicken fingers with an almond flour and flax seed coating as well as pancakes with coconut flour and bananas. Making a few changes every day helped relieve my anxiety and ease into this new way of eating. My symptoms began to improve, which gave me the positive reinforcement and incentive to keep going, and surprisingly, I was beginning to enjoy it.

Over time, I began to slowly incorporate even more plant-based ingredients into my meals. On Taco Tuesday, I started adding in a bunch of veggie or bean side dishes into the family meal and nobody noticed. Instead of just meat and cheese, I started roasting some cauliflower and sweet potatoes with paprika and cumin to use as a filler. I made some rice, black beans, extra guacamole, sautéed onions, peppers, and mushrooms to add to our burritos and bowls. When it comes to making a creamy cumin-lime sauce, I made it with a vegan sour cream, because it tastes the same anyway. These extras took the focus off the meat as the primary ingredient. Gradually, I prepared less meat and, sure enough, was amazed when there were some leftovers. This strategy is also incredibly helpful when trying to cook for people in various stages of transition or not in transition at all. If your spouse or child doesn't have the slightest interest in eating plant-based, they can still enjoy the benefit of a great meal with lots of tempting new options!

BUSINESS BITE

One approach to implementing a successful transformation is "chunking it up" into phases. Mergers are a good example of this. It's impossible to blend all the operations completely on day one so we often roll out the implementation in three stages or "chunks." A transition plan to combine jobs, technology, processes, and physical space requirements are each mapped out in the plan. Not only does this allow employees to "digest" the change in smaller pieces, it also gives the organization time to test out some of the designs and adjust accordingly for the subsequent phases.

BEFORE YOU BITE

No matter how different your food plan is from the way you eat today, a transition plan will ease you into the change. Depending on your health and sense of urgency, don't be afraid to try something radically new! If you simply want to try on a few changes, like eating more leafy greens and fewer packaged snacks, try it out and see how you feel. Adjust the pace of your transition plan according to your "stomach" for change. If you have eaten a peanut butter and jelly sandwich every day for lunch for the past twenty years, you may not want to switch to a kale/quinoa salad with butternut squash, toasted almonds, and cranberries tomorrow. Maybe a switch to almond butter on wheat bread will do the trick for now. It's not a race if you never get to the finish line, whether you are the tortoise or the hare, just keep moving forward.

Here are a few instructions for completing your own personal transition plan.

Column 1: Food I Eat Today

Start by writing down anything you typically like to eat. Think about the foods and meals you want to change first. Start with one food or meal, and then move to another.

Column 2: Easy Change

Identify some easy ways to upgrade your meal, moving you closer to your food plan. *Adjust the pace to suit your needs. Add or substitute more personal best foods into the food you eat today. Consider cooking your food in a different way (i.e. without breading, sauté, grill or steam instead of frying). Consider substituting your favorite processed food with one containing fewer ingredients.*

Column 3: Next Change

How can you build on your initial change and take this to the next level? *Continue to identify and incorporate even more personal best foods into your meals. Further reduce the amount of processed foods in your meal. Create additional charts as you identify new goals.*

Review the sample provided to help create your own custom transition plan.

Food I Eat Today	Easy Change	Next Change
Chicken fingers	Chicken strips with almond flour/flax meal	Grilled chicken strips with tomato sauce dip
Bacon and cheese omelet	Turkey and cheese omelet	Turkey, cheese, pepper and mushroom omelet
Boxed mac n' cheese	Organic mac n' cheese without dyes and artificial ingredients	Mac n' cheese with cauliflower
White pasta with butter	Brown rice pasta with butter	Brown rice pasta with one vegetable, olive oil, and a sprinkle of parmesan cheese
Peanut butter and jelly sandwich	Almond butter and jelly sandwich	Almond butter and bananas on a rice cake
Boiled string beans	Stir fry string beans with teriyaki	Stir fry string beans, carrots, and brown rice
Steamed carrots	Roasted carrots with thyme	Roasted carrots with leek and fennel
Cheese puffs/ nacho chips	Corn chips with guacamole	Rice/nut cracker with hummus
Chocolate cream cookies	Chocolate covered almonds	Trail mix with dark chocolate chips
Romaine salad with carrots and cucumbers	Spinach salad with roasted beets and artichoke hearts	Arugula salad with fennel and grapefruit
Coffee with extra sugar and cream	Coffee with raw honey and cream	Coffee with raw honey and almond/ coconut milk

PERSONAL TRANSITION PLAN

Food I Eat Today	Easy Change	Next Change

No two transition plans are exactly alike. No matter what food and wellness plan you select, the pace will vary based on your sense of urgency and "stomach" for change. While a massive diet change all at once can jumpstart your health, making small but sustainable changes to your current eating habits can also make a big difference over time. Your transition plan may include a little bit of both. Maybe you gradually work up to eliminating dairy in its entirety but decide now to cut out sugary snacks completely. Your transition plan should reflect your own individual approach.

Simplify the Process

Organizations often streamline processes to save time and money. How can you think like a business and identify ways you can simplify the process of cooking and eating every day? Planning ahead is so important to ensure you are "meal ready" at all times. Some of my health coaching clients create a full meal plan for the entire week and find this extremely helpful. But some find it too hard to plan that far ahead and it just doesn't work for them. In either case, simply keeping a few basic recipes and ingredients on-hand at all times will enable you to make a simple, delicious, and nutritious meal anytime.

We found that over 30% of those we surveyed have skipped an event because they were worried they wouldn't have access to safe or appropriate food.

The food transition survey asked those transitioning to a new diet to improve their health, "What do you find difficult about following your dietary restrictions?" The number one response (over 40%) was, "Food is not available or cooked properly out (restaurants, social or work events)." In fact, we found that over 30% of those we surveyed have skipped an event because they were worried they wouldn't have access to safe or appropriate food. Let's address this issue first.

Plan or eat ahead If possible, try to call ahead before heading to a party or event to see what they are serving and if they can accommodate your dietary restrictions. Your discussion will vary depending on your relationship with the host. Is it your sister or cousin, a close friend, or perhaps your spouse's business associate? You may be surprised at who goes out of their way to make accommodations for you. Don't expect your host to understand all the details of what you can and can't eat. Politely explain it as simply as possible. In the case of an allergy, express the severity and explain that, with some precaution, it's quite manageable.

Recently, my niece, who just moved into her first home, hosted Thanksgiving dinner this year. I was so incredibly touched when she made a special gluten-free mushroom stuffing just for my son and I. Cooking for others is such a gesture of love, and when someone goes out of their way to cook something special to support your health, it's very touching.

If you are headed out and have no idea what the food situation is, just eat ahead of time. You don't want to get caught at a work event or holiday party absolutely starving. Your risk of eating a trigger food is high, so try to avoid setting yourself up to fail by arriving with a full belly, ready to socialize.

We attended a large fundraising event in New York where many of the guests are actors and the menu is designed by a well-known celebrity chef. I thought for sure they would have a gluten-free option to accommodate this crowd, especially when the ticket price alone could feed an entire army of gluten-free soldiers. To my surprise, they were completely unprepared. After a bit of a scuffle, a plate of five vegetables arrived in front of me and dessert was a treat of sliced strawberries. I was starving and inevitably drank too much wine! Needless to say, we went out for dinner after it was over. Each year we attend, the choice improves but, just in case, I always eat something before heading out.

Shift Roles/Responsibilities This is a good time to discuss the roles and responsibilities in your home. You will be cooking a bit more so perhaps you could divide up the tasks of cleaning up, grabbing a few things at the store, or even taking on some basic cooking tasks such as washing or cutting up vegetables. Perhaps having more delicious food available in the house is an added incentive to your family! You are going to have to let go of a few things if you haven't already. You may take pride in winning the award for "perfect dishwasher loader," but maybe now is the time to let your kids and spouse take a crack at the title. The only kind of perfection you should strive for at this point is your version of "perfect health."

Save or Steal Time Imagine you have your heart set on a new giant television but don't have enough money to purchase it. You can save a little bit each week out of your current paycheck or you can take money out of another fund or expense you currently have. Think about making time to nourish and heal your body the same way. You have a certain amount of free time available that you can use, and/or you can take time away from something else you are doing to focus on your health (meal planning, cooking, wellness treatments, meditation, etc.). Everyone is busy and pressed for time, but I challenge you to find a little bit of time for yourself. Where will you save or steal the time from? Block time in your calendar to make this a daily priority. You are worth it.

Automate So many local grocery stores deliver for free over a certain purchase amount. Review the list of foods in your food plan and set up a standard delivery each week for the basics. Then, add a few extras as needed each week, depending on your schedule. You may find that you save money because you reduce the amount of impulse buying by not physically walking around the store. Have your shopping list available when setting up your weekly online order to help re-order items you run out of. Keep your shopping list on your phone so you're always prepared.

PERSONAL BITE

I am definitely a left-brained kind of girl. If you peek over my to-do lists, you will see an open box at the end of each task, and I don't feel satisfied until all the boxes are checked. Like a true consultant, no matter where I am or what I am doing, I always try to improve the process. Thank God my husband is also a management consultant because he can somewhat relate to this annoying habit. When things aren't operating smoothly from a restaurant to a hotel or even in my own house, I feel that it is my personal obligation to suggest a better way. I'm sure you, too, have been stuck in an unnecessary line or waited far too long for service due to poor operational practices. Yes, I'm the embarrassing one that offers up a better way.

With a clear food plan in place, I began to look for every opportunity possible to streamline the process of shopping and cooking. I started keeping a list of foods and ingredients to keep on hand and began to stock up on a few bulk items. I bookmarked and followed a few of my favorite social media food sites, nutrition websites, and recipe blogs.

I used the same basic spices for all my dishes to simplify and speed up my cooking. It's amazing what a few seasonings can do such as salt, pepper, onion powder, garlic powder, and any herb blend to prepare just about any main dish or side. Over time, I streamlined and standardized the prep process for almost every dish. It always started with chopping veggies, seasoning with the basics, and adding maybe one or two specialty flavors (i.e. ginger and soy sauce for Asian, cumin and chili powder for Mexican, basil and tomato sauce for Italian, and a fine herb blend and lemon for American dishes). After looking up a recipe idea online, I immediately skimmed through, looked for ways to simplify it, and adjusted the recipe to use only the personal best ingredients I had on-hand.

BUSINESS BITE

The tasks involved with simplifying the process of shopping and cooking to support a food and wellness transition were almost the same as the tasks required to plan a large-scale business or technology project. Use the following chart to think like a business change consultant and identify ways you can simplify the process!

Business TASK	Your TASK	Details
Assess current operations	Assess current eating habits	Compare the foods in your refrigerator and pantry to those in your new food plan. Update your shopping list and keep these foods in stock.
Identify technology needs	Identify cooking equipment needs	Do I need new pots, pans, knives, mixing bowls, cutting boards, peeler, etc. to help me in the kitchen?
Automate/ streamline business processes	Automate/simplify ways to shop and cook	Maintain online shopping lists and reminders, establish weekly grocery delivery of basic foods, subscribe to a few recipe blogs or sites that match your food plan or health problem. Download a few food/recipe apps on your phone. Organize using Pinterest or Evernote.
Address any culture changes. Identify change "champions" to rally support.	Address current food culture of my "tribe" of family, friends, and co-workers.	Is my tribe aligned with my new eating strategy? If not, how can I communicate with them to gain their support? Find and coordinate with the 1-2 people who "get it."
Adjust roles/ responsibilities	Who is responsible for what in my family?	How can I shift more responsibilities onto others to give me more time for shopping, cooking, and wellness?
Conduct training	What new skills do I need to support my new eating and wellness plan?	Should I take an online or local cooking class? How can I learn more about alternative wellness therapies (i.e. mindfulness, yoga)? Find local or online workshops.

Your Action List to Simplify the Process:

_____ ☐

_____ ☐

_____ ☐

_____ ☐

_____ ☐

_____ ☐

_____ ☐

_____ ☐

BEFORE YOU BITE

Take stock of your kitchen and your cabinets. How can you simplify the transition to a new way of eating and incorporate wellness practices into your routine? You may have the intent, but now you need to use the tools and tips to execute. Once you get in the habit of stocking your kitchen with the basics and keeping some fresh produce on hand, you will eventually be able to throw together a meal with whatever ingredients you have. I heard that... yes, you will, and I'm going to show you how.

Develop Job Aids In the change management world, "job aids" are a common practice. They are quick reference guides used to remind employees how to do something, especially when it is new to them. Think of a product code "cheat sheet" a cashier uses to checkout produce at the grocery store. Eventually, a seasoned cashier has all the codes memorized. But until then, a job aid is most helpful.

You, too, can use job aids to stay organized. Keep your personal best food list on-hand to simplify shopping. This is a great way to remind you of all the foods you can eat and enjoy. Many families with food allergies find that keeping lists of potentially harmful food ingredients on-hand is quite helpful for the first several months. After a while, you will know by heart exactly which foods and brands you can and can't eat.

Pantry List Keeping your pantry stocked is key to throwing together a quick meal at any time. Keep foods that you enjoy from your personal best food list on-hand, such as frozen or fresh fruits and vegetables. Post your pantry list on the inside of your cabinet or in your phone as a reminder. Refer to your specific food plan for a list of recommended pantry items such as beans, grains, nuts, seeds, and spices. Be careful to check all ingredient labels for any allergens. Remember that the longer the list of ingredients, the greater the chance the food isn't all that good for you.

Gluten-Free Tip Try this trick if you are a person with celiac transitioning to a gluten-free pantry, especially if not everyone in the family plans to become gluten-free. Use a Sharpie and mark every item in your pantry as "GF" or "NOT GF." Mark which stores your products came from so you remember for next time. This will be a big help until you can remember it all by heart.

Snack Menu It may sound funny, but I keep a snack menu on my fridge with over fifteen options for snacks that adhere to our family's eating style. We all find ourselves hungry between meals and grabbing the first thing we see may not be the best thing for us. Try to incorporate your personal best foods and identify at least ten snacks that you can grab or quickly prepare the next time you're hungry. The number one item on my snack menu is leftovers. My teenage son eats an entire leftover meal after school as a snack before we have dinner. Better that than a bunch of junk. Try cooking a little extra dinner and keep it on-hand for a delicious lunch or snack. Make a batch of grain or gluten-free muffins or granola bars to keep in the freezer to control how much sugar you are eating. A snack menu won't do you any good if you don't keep the ingredients in stock. Consider mixing up your snack list by adding a few new items every so often to encourage additional progress.

Many protein and granola bars are filled with sugar. When buying packaged snacks, keep in mind that 4 grams of sugar equals 1 teaspoon.

Cold Keeps Maintaining a good stock of quick go-to ingredients and to-go meals in the refrigerator and freezer will reduce frustration and keep you well fed. Buy fresh or frozen produce from your personal best list that can be used in a variety of recipes. It's also helpful to always keep a few prepared meals (previously made or purchased) in the freezer for when you're in a pinch. Most stores now carry frozen cooked grains (i.e. quinoa, brown rice) and, of course, frozen vegetables are great for a quick stir fry, grain bowl, or soup. Individually packed chicken breasts, turkey burgers, or veggie burgers are also great to have on-hand. Develop your own list of "cold keeps" using your food plan as a guide.

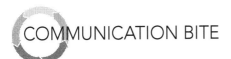

COMMUNICATION BITE

Continue learning and sharing from others along the way. This may uncover your co-worker's legendary vegetarian chili recipe or perhaps your neighbor is eternally grateful for your new snack menu. Don't be afraid of an uncomfortable conversation with your family about shared roles and responsibilities or an awkward discussion with your friend who keeps offering you off-limit foods, following it up with, "Oh, you can't have that, sorry." Stay aligned and keep close to those around you who "get it."

In the third bite to health, you commit to the change process by creating a detailed roadmap for your food and wellness plan. Channel the left-side of your brain to create a personal best food list and custom transition plan that honors your "stomach" for change. Use the methods provided to simplify the cooking process and prevent trigger food tragedies. Whether you type up a formal list in your phone or scribble notes on the back of a napkin, use your "job aids" as tools to keep you organized. Keep gaining knowledge and skills related to your food and wellness goals and look for ways to continue building upon your success.

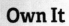

Own It

Create Food
Flexibility
—
Trial & Error
—
Burst the Barriers
to Change

4

CHAPTER SEVEN

4 Own It

Making changes to the way you eat today should start to feel a bit less forced and more natural. Trial and error puts you more in control of your food choices and allows you to perfect your understanding of how different foods impact your body. In this chapter, we will explore the idea of taking ownership to expand your transition plan even further. Imagine you are learning to speak Italian. One day, when you feel more comfortable with the language, you decide to test your skills by taking an Italian cooking class in Rome!

You will also use trial and error to perfect a set of recipe techniques aligned with your food plan. This will give you the "food flexibility" needed to prepare a variety of meals at any time.

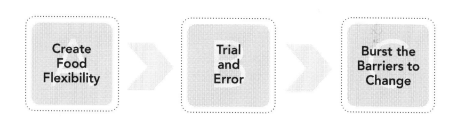

Create Food Flexibility → Trial and Error → Burst the Barriers to Change

Create Food Flexibility

This idea of "food flexibility" does not mean that some days you follow your food plan and some days you don't. What it does mean is that you the make the shift from individual recipes to mastering a few flexible cooking techniques. "Food flexibility" allows you to make a quick meal out of the ingredients you have on-hand. This skill will not only save you time and money but will keep you from going hungry and, I promise, it's quicker than take-out! Once you get in the habit of stocking your kitchen with the basics and keeping some fresh produce on-hand, you will be whipping up meals in no time.

The best way to create "food flexibility" is to KISS in the kitchen. Yes, a smack on the lips is exactly what you need! But when it comes to cooking and following a new food plan, I say, "Keep It Super Simple." Now is not the time to master every recipe from Julia Child or some complex blog post with ingredients you've never heard of and which are only useful in one dish. I often see clients burn out trying to make a complicated recipe every night, leaving fresh ingredients to rot in the drawer because they ran out of energy and time. Shopping for ingredients for one specific recipe can also be expensive, so focus on your personal best list of foods so they are re-usable for multiple meals.

When managing change, more choice is not always better. In fact, too many choices can be downright paralyzing. With a year-round availability of produce grown around the globe, your choices of ingredients and menu options have never been greater. As a result, we are overwhelmed with the idea of what to make for dinner and end up with the same few boring options.

There is a story about a small, poor Russian town where food availability was scarce. One day, residents in the town were given access to a full grocery store and given a stipend to purchase enough food for a week! They rushed into the store and, to their amazement, there were shelves lined with a variety of breads, cans of vegetables, and multiple kinds of meat and cheeses. However, after two hours of wandering around the store, most residents left with nothing. They were so overwhelmed with choice that it paralyzed them.

This may sound crazy, but now that I've settled into my eating habits, I think it's so much easier to shop and cook! Let me explain. It's like going into an enormous grocery store filled with food (or food-like substances) and being told that you can only eat food that is green. At first, this seems impossible and incredibly frustrating. But after your eyes get trained to quickly scan the isles, you begin to develop laser focus on only the green foods and can quickly grab them while going through store.

This is how I feel about eating food that is gluten-free, dairy-free, and minimally processed. I walk into a store with my food goggles on and go directly to the aisles with foods that I can eat. It's so easy to breeze by the many aisles of fake food because they don't match my food plan. This same strategy works when scanning the menu at a restaurant. It's like a game of Hide and Go Seek to identify the tasty foods that I can eat and enjoy. Eventually, I started shopping at smaller stores and co-ops in my area, which further reduced the time it took to shop for what I needed.

I believe that the overwhelming amount of choices we have has also contributed to the success of meal kit delivery services. Of course, the benefit of selecting and shipping ingredients is a time-saver, but I wonder if the real value is in limiting your choice as to what to make. Nobody complains about chopping and cooking or even cleaning up once the choice is selected for you.

Using Cookbooks I find one of the biggest problems with diet and healthy cookbooks is that they don't account for how you eat today. Think about it: How many recipes do you use in each cookbook? A few, maybe? Imagine you are a simple eater and a new diabetes diagnosis forces you to change your eating. You grab a cookbook but realize that you are not going to make balsamic figs with goat cheese as a snack on day one. Authors use their own personal favorite foods and eating style as a basis for their cookbook and it most likely doesn't match up exactly with yours. As you continue to get more comfortable substituting ingredients, you will not only make long-lasting changes to your eating habits but also get a lot more use out of all your cookbooks!

Too many recipe choices can be paralyzing, but too few is limiting. Focus on a set of ten basic yet flexible recipe techniques that you can use all the time. I still try new recipes occasionally, but my tried and true base is small enough to keep me sane while large enough to incorporate all my personal best foods into a variety of meals.

So many recipes use the same cooking method but simply change up a few ingredients to make it seem more complicated. Whether you have never cooked a meal in your life or you are a trained chef, once you master the basic processes, you are able to make a variety of meals. Add just one new ingredient or spice and, voila, a new dish is born! I rarely make the same meal twice because I never have the same fresh produce in the fridge. If you can chop, you can cook something new.

For example, on Thursday nights, I look at what's left in my produce drawer and decide how to mix it together to make a meal. This typically includes a rice bowl, stir fry, or soup with the leftover produce and anything else in my pantry (i.e. artichoke hearts, sundried tomatoes). For added protein, I throw in some lentils, beans, or defrost a chicken breast or ground turkey from the freezer. This is a great way to save money by using up all your ingredients, so nothing gets thrown away. Your meal also makes a great leftover to have on-hand throughout the weekend (if there is anything left)!

> **Food flexibility allows you to make a quick meal with whatever ingredients you have on-hand.**

Your level of food flexibility will also encourage you to try new ingredients because you aren't sticking to the exact same recipe all the time. If you like broccoli and cauliflower, try Romanesco, a light green combination of both vegetables. Try changing the color of your favorite food, like purple broccoli or orange cauliflower. Eating foods with a variety of colors gives your body a variety of nutrients, so simply changing the color of your food promotes change and improves your health!

Sample Top 10 Recipe Techniques Here is a sample of ten simple recipe techniques that can be made with a variety of personal best foods. To customize your own top 10 list, search for very simple but flexible recipe styles that are aligned with your food plan. Use trial and error as you go to adjust flavors and ingredients to make the recipe your own. My sample list is primarily for dinner, but once you get the hang of it, create a top 10 for lunch and breakfast, too.

Once you have the confidence to cook with a set of 10 recipe techniques that adhere to your food plan, then go ahead and try a more complicated recipe using out of the ordinary ingredients or spices. You may just find yourself adjusting that recipe, too!

10 Recipe Techniques

1 Simple Stir Fry
Mix any veggies, nuts, and/or protein* over (cauliflower) rice and toss with ginger and teriyaki sauce.

2 Mexican Fiesta (taco, burrito, bowl)
Use taco seasoning to flavor protein*, roasted veggies, steamed sweet potatoes, and/or sautéed peppers, onions, zucchini, and mushrooms. Add salsa to a side of rice. Try a side of beans, guacamole, or cumin-lime vegan sour cream sauce.

3 Custom Frittata
Add eggs to any sautéed veggies and bake for a meal anytime.

4 Easy Veggie Soup
Sauté any veggies and protein*. Add broth, beans, and herbs to taste.

5 Flexi-Veggie Pasta
Sauté any veggies and protein*. Add to cooked (GF) pasta with a little cooking water to make a sauce or add a jar of your favorite tomato sauce. Add a splash of citrus or vinegar to balance the flavor.

6 Basic Risotto
Follow directions on package and add roasted or sautéed veggies and/or protein*.

7 Grain & Roasted Veggie Bowl
Mix and match your favorite veggies, grains, beans, and protein*.

8 Lettuce Wraps
Sauté any veggies, grains, beans, and protein*. Add water chestnuts for crunch, and toss with rice wine vinegar, soy sauce, and lime juice.

9 Kitchen Sink Salad
Mix anything you have on-hand including roasted veggies, nuts, seeds, and proteins*. Experiment with simple salad dressings.

10 Red or White Chili (meat, veggie, or both)
Use chili powder and taco seasoning to flavor protein*, beans and/or sweet potatoes. Add a variety of veggies and canned tomatoes (for red) or broth (for white).

*protein may include any meat, fish, tofu, tempeh, etc.

Note: If you must jump quickly to a new food plan or have identified several new allergies all at once, you can immediately go from identifying your personal best foods to creating your top 10 recipe techniques. For example, Karen was recently diagnosed with Lyme disease and decided to try a new diet by eliminating all grains, tree nuts, dairy, and legumes immediately. She quickly developed her "go-to" set of ten flexible recipes to help plan her meals. Karen went from feeling overwhelmed to feeling food flexible!

BUSINESS BITE

Businesses often identify and focus their time and resources on a handful of key processes that make up most of the work. Think of a customer service call center. Most calls that come in fall into a few categories, resulting in a common recording: "Press 1 for [X]," and, "Press 2 for [Y]," etc. Staff and training is focused on handling these primary calls. Occasionally, a call will come in that requires someone with a specific skillset or knowledge base. It doesn't make sense to train the entire customer service center on every possible call scenario. These specific calls are transferred to a small set of employees trained in that specific area. This maximizes efficiency but also improves the quality of service to the customers as they are matched quickly with a representative who is well versed to handle their request.

PERSONAL BITE

I decided to apply the business approach above to further streamline the cooking process. I began to home in on a set of ten very simple recipe techniques that were flexible enough to incorporate a variety of my personal best foods and staple ingredients. I also happen to love all the dishes that these techniques allow me to create and I didn't need to become a professional chef to do this.

Occasionally, I enjoy making a special recipe and will shop for a few ingredients outside my normal staples (like pad Thai with crushed peanuts and bean sprouts). I also enjoy meals outside of my normal repertoire out at a restaurant. For example, I don't make a whole branzino as part of my weekly or monthly routine, but I do enjoy this if dining at a nice restaurant. In other words, "Table for 2" and, "Press 3 for branzino."

BEFORE YOU BITE

Now, I know what you're saying to yourself and I hear it a lot: "I just can't throw together a meal. I must follow a specific recipe!" If that is the case, then find one or two simple recipe techniques (i.e. stir fry or grain bowl) and perfect them first. Then practice substituting a few personal best ingredients you have on-hand. Eventually, you should settle into a set of around ten techniques that work for you. Then you can begin using vegetables that are local or in season. This will give you the flexibility you need to make a hundred different meals on any given night, depending on what's in your kitchen. Take a moment and identify your top 10 recipe techniques.

10 Recipe Techniques

1 _____

2 _____

3 _____

4 _____

5 _____

6 _____

7 _____

8 _____

9 _____

10 _____

Trial and Error

When it comes to change, no one can expect perfect results on the first try. Over 30% of people in the food transition survey reported that trial and error was important when transitioning to a diet with food restrictions. Give your body some time to adjust to your food plan. Be honest about what works and what doesn't and adjust accordingly. Taking the time to evaluate your approach and your progress thus far is critical. This allows you to expand upon the things you are doing well and adjust the things that just aren't working. Now might also be a good time to try a new wellness practice and test the results.

There are times we must look at the quality of our life and weigh the benefits and consequences of eating a certain way. If after a while, your food plan seems to be taking over your life in an unnecessary or negative way, it might be time to re-evaluate. **The goal is to create a perfect balance between your level of effort and the health results you want to achieve.** I promise you will soon get to a point where you want to eat a certain way just to feel great versus feeling forced to do so. Your personal eating strategy will become second nature soon after.

> *"I had 3 sinus surgeries to remove polyps and chronic infections. Two weeks after going dairy-free, I found relief and astounded my doctor."*
> — Anonymous Survey Response

You may also be surprised to find that the "healthy" food or drink in your plan isn't agreeing with you. For example, I have found that drinking kombucha (a fermented tea) helps with digestion and heals my gut. I also have seen others who feel incredibly bloated from the drink but keep drinking it because it's "good for them." Perhaps drinking it in small amounts or less often will have a greater impact. If you notice something isn't right, don't be afraid to admit it and make a change.

Do a little dance Eventually, you become fluent in your body's language and you reach a mode where you have a strong understanding of how it reacts to a variety of different foods. When tweaking your plan, you may find yourself "doing a little dance" where you strictly avoid some foods while enjoying others in moderation, accepting the minor consequences. The same applies to your wellness practices. You may find the 5-minute mindfulness practice helpful but don't necessarily need to listen to the 20-minute guided meditation every night before bed. Perhaps you saw some benefits from a salt room or sauna when struggling with your sinuses but decided to save a little money for a lymphatic massage next month. As the CEO of your health, you are responsible for setting priorities, managing operations, and approving the budget!

Here are a few examples of clients "doing a little dance" with their food and health:

Suzie suffered with interstitial cystitis for 26 years. After following a paleo plan (coupled with acupuncture and stress management) for over a year with a lot of success, she shifted to a less strict primal diet, which included adding legumes and eggs back in as tolerated. She settled on an eating plan that matched her desired amount of change within her current lifestyle and which provided her with maximum health benefits.

Allison followed the GAPS diet[1] to alleviate symptoms caused by her ulcerative colitis. She felt amazing and her symptoms disappeared after a year. She began to eat gluten again and then, after a stressful event at work, her symptoms re-appeared. She found blood in her stool and had diarrhea just like before. Allison went back on an adjusted version of the GAPS diet and eventually found a happy medium that kept her symptom-free but isn't as restrictive.

[1]The GAPS diet is for naturally treating chronic inflammatory conditions in the digestive tract. A great resource is the *Gut and Psychology Syndrome*, by Natasha Campbell-McBride, M.D.

Through trial and error, you will eventually settle into a way of eating that balances your food choices with your quality of life and the benefits you want to achieve. Some struggle trying to find that balance. Most people give up completely at this point, especially if they jumped into their food plan 100% on day one without a structured plan of action. They eventually run out of self-control.[14] Instead of throwing in the towel altogether, just slow down and readjust. If you go on vacation and go off the deep end, don't let that hijack all your progress thus far.

I see many people give up on their food plan, even if they are enjoying dramatic results. In this case, just remember that it doesn't have to be all or nothing (unless you have a food allergy). Doing your best and feeling good about it beats perfection with misery every time. You will get there eventually. Just be kind to yourself and don't forget to reward yourself along the way for all your hard work!

My friend had pancreatic cancer and he tried a variety of food plans throughout his battle that made a huge difference in extending his life. He tried an all raw food diet for a while but, eventually, it got in the way of his quality of life (hanging out with friends, visiting family) and he modified it. He taught me that everyone has their limit and balance is key. I am so grateful for his insight and for our many conversations about the power of food. He has inspired me in so many ways to do the work I do today. Remember that you know your body best so be a good listener and you will find the right balance of food, health, and happiness.

PERSONAL BITE

I made significant changes to my diet because I needed to kickstart my healing to address my symptoms quickly. I ate (almost) completely grain-free and dairy-free for a few months and used trial and error along the way. I tried a variety of dairy-free ice creams and settled on a tie between a coconut milk strawberry and a cashew milk vanilla that were my favorites. I tried every non-dairy creamer on the market and finally found one made from a pea protein that is amazing. After a while, though, as my symptoms subsided,

I realized that eating grain-free left me feeling hungry and I began to look a bit scrawny. I decided to add some gluten-free grains back in, like brown rice and quinoa. I still enjoy the health benefits, but this adjustment helped me feel and look better. As I continued to detox, the numbness and tingling in my legs continued to decline, the number of sinus infections decreased, and I even saw an improvement in a bladder condition that I found out was also related to my nervous system. Overall, I settled into a new normal with my eating habits and it felt pretty darn good.

To this day, I "do a little dance" to create the right balance between my eating habits and my health. While nobody eats perfectly all the time (maybe Giselle and Tom Brady), I have settled on a nice balance of food choices that keep my symptoms at bay while maintaining a quality of life that suits me. Sometimes there is a trade-off. While eating meat-free improves my digestion, I find that just a little bit of chicken or fish keeps me feeling satisfied (for now). Equipped with this knowledge, I often consult with my body and adjust the plan as time goes on.

BUSINESS BITE

Successful businesses adept at change also use the trial and error method in a concept called "test and learn." This is quite useful when testing a new product offering to their customers. Telephone service representatives may offer a new product during a routine phone call with a smaller segment of customers or perhaps limit the offer to certain times of the day. This allows the company to gain valuable insight and test customer interest levels before rolling the product out nationwide.

Imagine calling up a nationwide glass company to fix your broken windshield. During the service call, they ask if you would be interested in having your car detailed during your glass repair. It won't take long for them to gather enough data to wane interest levels before offering it to all customers.

Every transformation project takes time out to assess the initial approach and evaluate the progress made. It's easy to keep charging ahead without taking the much-needed time required to evaluate what's working and what needs to be fine-tuned or thrown out completely. This is the role of the "project management team" on a change transformation initiative. These dedicated resources are focused on tracking progress and facilitating changes as quickly as possible when needed.

BEFORE YOU BITE

How can you do a little dance to find the right balance of food choice and quality of life? Try to stay motivated along the way and reward yourself for taking such good care of your body. Continue using trial and error to test foods and brands that you enjoy. Some get addicted to feeling great and decide to stick to their food plan 100% from here on out. Others say that the simple idea of never eating a certain type of food ever again for the rest of their life sounds too scary. Pick an approach that resonates with your personality and vision for health.

Prioritize choices to find balance. There are times when a substitute for a favorite food is almost as good as the original. For example, there are so many delicious dairy-free ice creams on the market. Why sacrifice your goals when there are other options available? Other times, you may decide that a little goes a long way. For example, our favorite local artisan pizza place has the best gluten-free crust but the worst dairy-free cheese. So, occasionally, instead of no cheese, I'll get a gluten-free pizza with regular cheese. We don't go out for pizza very often, so when I do have it, I really enjoy it. I call this the **"last man standing."** It's the one food that you simply cannot give up 100% (if you don't absolutely have to). The amount of change required for the benefit is simply not worth it.

Progress Evaluation Employees have performance evaluations, so should your food and wellness plan. What have you learned about your food preferences and restrictions using trial and error? Take some time to reflect upon what's working and what might need some adjustment. Resist the temptation to keep charging ahead with your plan without carefully evaluating your approach and progress. As always, be honest and remember you are in a "no-judgement" zone. Be kind to yourself, especially when you decide to eat something not in your plan. The natural consequences are far worse than any guilt trip, so don't bother. You are making progress overall and that's what counts. Keep up the good work!

Answer the following questions to help assess your progress and adjust where needed.

How is the transition to your new eating habits going on a scale of 1 to 10? Why did you assign this rating?

_____

_____

What are 3 things that are working well in your food and wellness plan and how can you expand upon them?

_____

_____

What are 3 things that you would like to change? How?

_____

_____

Are you making the amount of progress you hoped for at this point? Why or why not?

_____

_____

Burst the Barriers to Change

What might still be getting in your way of progress? Recognizing your barriers to change is important and removing them is critical to your success. Barriers will always exist, but we must not use them as excuses, rather opportunities to rise above and conquer them. There are some barriers that are internal (i.e. not prioritizing your time properly) and some that are external (i.e. the availability of food at a work function). We have addressed many solutions to these barriers throughout the book. At this point in the change, you have planned for as much as possible, but a few obstacles may remain or may have popped up along the way. Now is the time to address them.

PERSONAL BITE

One of my biggest change barriers was self-inflicted. I realized that I was procrastinating and continuing to put everyone else's needs above my own. On a typical crazy morning, handcrafted organic lunches were made for the kids, the kitchen was somewhat cleaned up, and everything was ready to go. However, I often ran out of the mere ten minutes needed to start my day with an intention, prepare my own breakfast, or take my supplements. I call it the Cinderella syndrome. Everyone was ready for the ball, but I was left to finish my chores. After a while of using "lack of time" as an excuse for my lack of progress, I began to wonder, "How is it possible that only ten minutes is getting in the way of my progress?"

Was I the barrier to my own change? Was I self-sabotaging my own progress, and if so, why? Did I really think that I was a bad mother if I put my own health needs first? No way. After all the work I had put in thus far, this idea was not acceptable. So, I re-focused my health vision and how important it was to me and re-committed to the plan. I set the alarm 10 minutes earlier and took care of my own needs first. It reminded me of when the airline tells you to put the mask on yourself first before giving oxygen to those you love. It can feel a little selfish at first, but necessary for survival. So, I tightened the strap and took the first breath.

BUSINESS BITE

Businesses often struggle with their own barriers to change and need to be prompted to think creatively to solve the problem. When I facilitated group design sessions, I often shared this story with the group to challenge their thinking and develop creative, "out of the box" ideas.

A young mother cooks a roast every Sunday, and prior to placing it in the roasting pan, she cuts off the front and back of the roast. When her child asked, "Mommy, why do you cut the ends off the roast?" her reply is simply, "I don't know. That's how Nana taught me, and I always do it this way." Out of curiosity, the child went to the grandmother and asked the same question. The grandmother answered in a similar fashion, "That's how your great-grandmother taught me to do it." Luckily, the great-grandmother was still alive, and so the child called her up, hoping for a better answer. The great-grandmother replied, "Oh dear, when I cooked our Sunday roast, we never had a pan quite big enough to fit such a large piece of meat, so I would cut the ends off a bit before putting it in the pan and into the oven."

Businesses also get stuck in a rut of "because that's how we've always done it" instead of looking for the root cause of the problem and how to fix it. Our goal is to challenge ourselves by thinking creatively and to keep asking, "Why?" Who would have thought that the best advice comes from modeling a four-year-old?

BEFORE YOU BITE

What barriers are you faced with? Even after all the planning and early success, are there a few things that keep getting in your way? Perhaps you still find yourself shopping, ordering, cooking and eating a certain way out of habit. Whether your barriers are self-inflicted, within your control or outside of your influence, what are they and how can you think creatively to address them?

Here are a few common examples of change barriers I often hear with clients:

> It's too expensive to eat this way.

> It's hard to eat this way with my long work hours.

> I eat out a lot for work and don't have a lot of options.

> My kids' schedules make home cooking difficult.

> My social life with friends revolves around meals that are not aligned with my food plan.

> None of my extended family eats remotely close to my food plan and my spouse is also a bad influence.

The list goes on and on. But for every barrier, you can brainstorm at least three potential solutions. Barriers to change are just excuses not to get the change started. For every barrier that exists, there is a way to rise and hurdle over it or simply break through.

Here are a few possible solutions to common change barriers:

1 Use the bulk section of stores to purchase grains and other dry goods at a discount.

2 Set up a standard weekly delivery of basic personal best groceries each week with free shipping.

3 Batch cook ingredients (quinoa, rice, roasted vegetables) to use throughout the week to save money and time.

4 Make a batch of healthy muffins or granola bars and freeze for a quick snack.

5 Eat before you go to a party or work event.

6 Find and suggest a new restaurant to your friends that caters to dietary restrictions.

7 Pack your lunch and bring plenty of snacks to all day children's outings.

8 Have ingredients in the freezer for five meals that are faster than take-out.

9 Bring a new dish in your food plan to your friend or family's dinner.

10 Scan the menu at a work dinner to find acceptable foods, then ask the chef to combine them into a meal that adheres to your food plan.

CHANGE BARRIERS

What is getting in the way of achieving your health vision and what are some possible solutions?

Potential Barriers	Possible Solutions

COMMUNICATION BITE

Take advantage of the group you "teamed up" with early on and solicit their input to create your list of ten recipe techniques. Remember that a few failures are not only expected but an important part of the change process. Share war stories of lessons learned through trial and error. Change is never perfect and it helps to be genuine when going through the process. I found that pretending everything was easy during the transition caused more stress than it was worth. Be authentic and you will find that people who care about you are genuinely interested in supporting you.

In the fourth bite to health, you find yourself taking ownership of your food and wellness plan. You settle into a new normal and the process of shopping and cooking feels a lot more natural. As you establish a level of food flexibility, you can feel more comfortable experimenting with a variety of new foods. Through trial and error, you establish a much clearer understanding of your body's language and how different foods make you feel. As a result, you are empowered to create a balance between food choice, health, and quality of life. Be honest about the things that may still be getting in your way and have the courage to address them. Gaining strength, both physically and mentally, you now have a renewed sense of control and confidence.

**Reinvent
Health**

Celebrate
Success
—
Raise the Bar
—
Spread
the Love

5

CHAPTER EIGHT

5 Reinvent Health

You have made it to the final step! Now is time to reflect and take the much-needed time to celebrate all the progress you have made thus far in your health! Feeling better is the best reward of all! Now an expert in your body's language, you find it easy to diagnose a mild headache, heartburn, a new hive or rash on your face. You can quickly identify the potential food culprit, test your theory, and remove it if needed.

Consider applying all that you have learned to make additional changes in your food and wellness plan and improve your health even further. The second time through The 5 Bites to Health is so much easier because you are more comfortable with the process and with change itself. Can you even remember how it felt when you first embarked on this journey? What may seem like second nature to you now certainly didn't feel that way back then. Looking back, what do you wish you knew? Pay it forward and share your insights to help someone else the way others helped you.

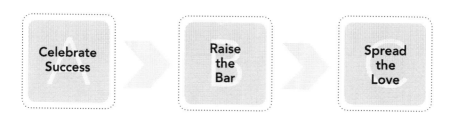

Celebrate Success → Raise the Bar → Spread the Love

Celebrate Success

Before you grab the champagne glasses to celebrate your success, let's first take a moment... I know, here I go again with the go slow to go fast. But let's take a moment to thank your body. Thank your body for speaking to you and showing you how to properly care for it. Show your body that you are now an active listener. You have gained a newly found respect for the job your body does and will not take it for granted again. Think of this as the toast at a wedding. There is a reason the toast comes in the beginning of the night and it's not because people are mostly sober then (although that probably doesn't hurt). The toast forces everyone to stop and reflect. I believe the toast is a form of mindfulness that sets the tone for the evening. Picture when the reception room becomes completely quiet and guests all take time to share their love and gratitude for the couple and celebration ahead. What a wonderful custom. Why don't we have toasts more often?

Positive psychology research indicates that gratitude is strongly and consistently associated with greater happiness.[15] The mere act of reflecting on all that you have to be thankful for contributes to your overall wellbeing. It turns out those with a glass half-full mentality are obviously more positive and they could be healthier, too. Practicing gratitude and thanking your body for all it does could be the cheapest but most effective medicine around, and you don't need a prescription to get it.

PERSONAL BITE

I used to be so anxious about getting a viral infection, so fearful that my numbness and tingling throughout my body would escalate to something else. OCD behaviors such as wiping down door knobs, steering wheels, and water bottles, or getting annoyed when someone picked up my coffee cup or water glass became common. But I can now relax and celebrate how far I've come. The final test occurred recently when I was a lector at mass on Sunday. I had to take a sip of wine from the chalice after the priest and all the eucharistic ministers had done so before me. While they do wipe the chalice and turn it before each person takes a sip, I've always declined, practically running off the alter. But last week, as I wrote the last chapter of my book, I took a sip of wine in triumph and remained healthy enough to tell the story.

I found that the more appreciative I was of my body and all it did for me, the happier and better I felt overall. It seems my body and I now have a new understanding. We take care of each other and, as a result, I don't have to worry so much about getting sick. I guess you could say it has my back.

BUSINESS BITE

Businesses often celebrate success. They demonstrate gratitude to valued customers by providing them with special coupons or credits toward additional purchases. I am noticing more opportunities for customers to provide specific feedback and recommend rewards to company employees. For example, after a recent delivery from Pottery Barn, I received an email soliciting feedback on the delivery person's service, asking for a rating between 1 to 5 stars. The next question asked: "If you think we should reward John for great service, simply select one of the options below: a) High five b) Thank you note or c) Gift card. Of course, I recommended a gift card! This earned Pottery Barn much goodwill and earned John a gift card. Everybody is a winner!

Recognizing and celebrating an employee's special talent or hosting a party for members of a recent change project creates so much goodwill and respect within the organization. It reminds me of a favorite quote from *The Sidur Sim Shalom, Prayer Book for Peace*: "We have come into being to praise, to labor, and to love."[16] If more businesses and individuals can follow this advice, we can all share in the rewards.

BEFORE YOU BITE

To celebrate your own success, take some time to show gratitude for your body and celebrate your healing. Even if you were never sick to begin with, through this process, you have most likely established a better relationship with your body that will serve you well. As the person giving the toast at a wedding, you, too, can bring others in to "raise their glass" and share in your success and happiness. Thank others for their love and encouragement throughout your transition. Consider writing a note to someone who was particularly supportive and perhaps the brunt of your complaints during difficult times. Thanking your body and your tribe for their support is the best way to get this celebration started! Get in the habit of practicing gratitude every day and, I promise, your body will thank you right back.

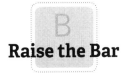

Raise the Bar

Are you ready to build on the momentum and "raise the food bar" again? It's like having a one-year-old who is finally sleeping through the night and you decide to get pregnant again! If you're up for it, perhaps remove other top allergens to see how you feel. Gradually, at a pace that feels right, you can remove and add new foods into your diet until your health vision is a reality. Be careful not to take on more food challenges than you can handle at different points in your life.

When you raise the bar, you will notice that the second time through the change is so much easier. Imagine you have lost power in your home during a storm and it's 9:00 p.m. The first time this happens, you are shocked and wonder, "What do I do now?" Eventually, you stumble around for some flashlights and candles, adjust your bedtime routine, and go to bed. You remember to stock up on a few items, like batteries and a back-up phone charger, in case this happens again. A few weeks later, another storm hits and bam! No power. But this time, you aren't very worried. You quickly find the items you prepared earlier and kick into gear. You are confident that all will be okay because you have been through it once before.

Once you are feeling better and in more of a maintenance mode, you may decide instead of raising the bar, to lower it and loosen up on part of your food plan. Over 17% of people in the food transition survey said they snuck foods back into their diet when symptoms subsided. Maybe you are exhausted from too much change too quickly and decide to ease up. For example, maybe you tried to go 100% sugar-free, but after 6 months, decided that a little honey in your coffee and an occasional piece of dark chocolate feels just fine. You may also inadvertently slip back into denial and test your trigger foods all over again to see if they do, in fact, still affect you. It's like having that last glass of wine. Why am I so shocked when it makes me feel so terrible the next day?

If you add foods back in and don't get an immediate reaction, proceed with caution and make a mental note. You may not immediately start throwing up or have diarrhea like a person with a severe allergy might. But after eating your trigger food a few times here and there, you may accumulate the toxin in your body which eventually causes symptoms to appear all over again, and perhaps worse than before. Now, if you're lucky, you may find that you can occasionally enjoy a food that had once been considered a "trigger" but can now be tolerated in moderation.

> *I repeatedly tried to reintroduce [trigger food] thinking I was "better." I am now resigned to never touching it again.*
>
> — *Anonymous Survey Responder*

PERSONAL BITE

I have always loved sugar and carbs. Give me a bag of candy fish, a bagel, or a soft pretzel and a sugary yogurt and I was in heaven. After my original food transition, taking gluten and dairy out of my diet, I began to see much success and my symptoms were alleviated. I stopped eating junk candy but enjoyed a little dark chocolate once in a while. However, I did not realize just how much sugar was still creeping into my diet. After adding it all up over an entire day, I realized that sugar was going to be the next bar raised. I already transitioned to a strawberry almond yogurt away from my favorite cherry Greek yogurt, and this was a great first step. But once I focused on reducing my sugar intake, I found an amazing new plant-based yogurt made with coconut cream, pili nuts, and root vegetables that produces the same creamy texture and delicious taste. I also began buying the plain versions of other non-dairy yogurts and adding some granola, nuts, and dried fruits, or a little honey into it. This is how I raised the bar to reduce the amount of sugar in my diet, and I used a personal transition plan to make small changes from how I was eating to achieve my goals.

What's next on the bar for me? I would like to test out the benefits of an intermittent fasting program. But for right now, I'm good.

BUSINESS BITE

Successful businesses are often those where change is inherently part of the culture. Companies must continue to develop the next idea and transform themselves repeatedly to stay relevant and survive in an ever-changing marketplace. Facebook is a great example. The website was initially developed to connect classmates and has evolved into a global networking powerhouse. They now host discussion forums for interest groups, businesses, and education. Facebook has become a major platform for marketing and sales of new and used products. My guess is that they aren't going to ever stop changing to keep up with customer demands, although they may soon be implementing new regulations.

"In life, change is inevitable. In business, change is vital."
—*Warren G. Bennis*

BEFORE YOU BITE

Think about where you are on the bar and what your next goal is. Even if you choose not to raise the bar now, at least identify the area you would like to address next once you have the stomach for it.

What I find funny is that your lowest bar—the food you won't eat—may change without you realizing it. Twenty years ago, I would have eaten a McDonald's cheeseburger once in a blue moon without thinking about it.

Now, I wouldn't even eat a bowl of regular pasta. Which foods would you not eat in a million years now? How has this changed throughout your own transformation?

SAVOR IT: Stop and reflect upon the amount of change you have endured thus far. Are you motivated by your progress and ready to take on more? Are you a little burned out and need a break? Or are you like Goldilocks and everything feels just right?

raising the food bar

Diet almost completely comprised of:

Only organic whole foods such as fruits, vegetables, beans, nuts, seeds, plant or pasture-raised protein.

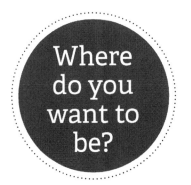

Where do you want to be?

Mostly whole and organic foods low in sugar. Occasionally eat processed foods (with minimal number of ingredients).

About half of food is processed and half is whole food based.

Mostly processed foods with some whole foods added into meals.

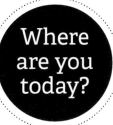

Where are you today?

Almost completely processed foods, many high in sugar (frozen meals, pizza, fast food, donuts, breads, cookies, crackers, cereal, protein bars, foods with corn syrup, enriched flour, artificial ingredients, etc.).

Raising the Food Bar Notes:

_____

_____

_____

_____

_____

Spread the Love

The way you know you are through a food change is when you begin to help someone else going through a similar struggle. What a rewarding feeling and quite cathartic as well! You may look back at your journey and feel a sense of pride. It's like renovating a kitchen. It was hell going through it, but the result was totally worth it!

Sharing your experience, the good and bad, is healing for you as well. It's a "been there, done that" mentality. Our memory is often short to block out unpleasant times (i.e. that 20-hour road trip wasn't THAT bad with the kids… oh, it was worse). Be careful not to make it sound like "it was no big deal to give up sugar for a year" because it is a big deal and you will come off as insincere. Acknowledge the struggle and encourage others with something like, "If I can give up sugar, anyone can!" Much better.

Have empathy for someone else going through the same food change process. How rewarding to turn a face filled with anxiety into a relieved smile! You will surprise yourself as to how much you have learned in your journey, even if you still have more changes to make. The process of reflecting on "what you wish you knew" and sharing your lessons learned with someone eager to listen is quite cathartic.

You can't save the world. After you have transformed your own eating habits and your health, you are living proof of the power of food! The hardest part of having this new knowledge is that when you see others who could benefit from a similar transformation, they may not be ready for the change. You will hear someone talk about their painful symptoms or a new diagnosis and you want to scream and tell them how food and other healing treatments can change their life!

Just as you asked not to be judged during your own transformation, respect others and do not try to change their mind if they are not ready. The last thing they want to hear is you preaching on a soapbox, and they will immediately resist everything you say. I've had to bite my tongue so many times, it's amazing I can still speak. We tell executives to "lead by example," and that's the best advice for you, too. Let them see what you're doing and how amazing you feel. Tell them you are here if and when they are ready to talk.

PERSONAL BITE

I have always been energized by sharing information to make someone else's life easier or better in some way. That's probably what drove me to consulting in the first place. Now, as a health coach, I get to "spread the love" all the time. I finally understand what it means to marry what you are knowledgeable and skilled in with something you are truly passionate about. I love and learn from my clients all the time. I feel a great sense of pride in guiding them on their health journey and witnessing their transformation. With a shared sense of trust, we keep each other motivated to stay healthy every day.

BUSINESS BITE

Customers value the idea of "giving back" and are directing their spending dollars to companies that do too. Toms was an early adopter to incorporate service directly into their business strategy. For every pair of shoes purchased, a pair of shoes is donated to a child in need as part of their "One for One" program. Bombas is another great example. They are a sock company that was created to address the huge need for socks in homeless shelters. A goal of one million donated socks has quickly turned into a donation of over eight million pairs with the live counter on their website raising by the second. If we are grateful for what we have, it becomes much easier to "spread the love" to others. Now more businesses than ever are finding a way to do just that and customers are literally buying into it.

BEFORE YOU BITE

Your new health story is a revised edition that is both interesting and helpful to others. You will inevitably cross paths with someone who shares a similar food and health journey as you. Take some time to share "what you wish you had known" or share the top three things you learned to help ease their transition. If you pay it forward, so will they.

Just as you relied on specific discussion boards and feeds to answer your questions and gain support, take a moment to pop back on and answer a few questions for yourself. Be warned! The discussion boards can get very ugly with lots of judgment and negativity. Rise above it all and stay positive. If you see a need in an area that hasn't been covered, start a new page to share your knowledge in that area. If you are interested in this topic, chances are there are plenty of others who are, too.

Join a national or local community group in your health and wellness area to share your story and learn from others. For example, organizations like Beyond Celiac are conducting much needed research and compiling data for users to compare their experiences across a broader audience. Perhaps you are part of an online vegan group, such as Forks Over Knives, and would like to attend their annual conference. You may benefit from becoming a part of the American Diabetes Association and community. You have lots to share and plenty more to learn.

Consider attending a wellness workshop or explore becoming a health coach yourself! Ask yourself how else you can "spread the love" and share all you have learned to help others. You never know, the person you help may just inspire you to raise the bar yet again.

How can I share the love to help others?

COMMUNICATION BITE

Other people may notice that you have settled in to a "new normal" before you do. Perhaps you receive a compliment on how good you look, or your overall demeanor may appear a bit more relaxed. Ask, listen, and take advantage of others' observations on your transition. Like it or not, their honest and objective feedback may provide you with valuable insight on how to adjust your plan. Embrace your success by using all you have learned to support others. Someone else gave their precious time to help you and now it is your chance to pay it forward to someone else.

In the fifth and final bite, take the time to reflect on all you have accomplished thus far. You don't need to eat perfectly all the time or achieve all your health goals to reach this step in the change process. Whether you have decided to raise the bar yet again or if you have settled into a nice balance of food choices and health benefits, change has naturally become a part of your everyday life. For example, you may surprise yourself one afternoon by switching out your regular afternoon coffee with a new matcha tea latte!

You have gained some new superpowers throughout this process. You now have the power to interpret subtle messages from your body and have developed laser focus on what foods to look for both in the grocery store and on the restaurant menu. The best part of all is that you can use these powers for good (not evil, of course) by helping others.

Now that your new eating habits and cooking skills are on "auto pilot," you may wonder why it all seemed so hard before when it is all you know now. When looking back at how you used to eat, you probably don't miss it and you especially don't miss how you used to feel. Thank your body and show gratitude to those around you for supporting your transition. Now, let the party begin!

CHAPTER NINE

Beyond Food

Congratulations! You have made a significant impact on your health by changing your eating habits and incorporating a variety of wellness practices into your routine! The impact of different foods on your body is so much easier to detect and I'm sure you are continuing to learn new things about this relationship every day.

When you are ready, consider raising the bar yet again and go back through The 5 Bites to Health to implement other non-food changes for a total health transformation. Consider mixing up your exercise, mindfulness practice, non-toxic beauty and cleaning supplies, and swapping out clean pesticides for your home. I urge you to address these components one by one and, once again, respect your personal "stomach" for change to determine the right pace of change for you.

Practice change in non-food ways:

▶ Try a paraben-free shampoo

▶ Replace your deodorant with a non-aluminum version

▶ Change your workout

▶ Use a vinegar spray as a weed killer

▶ Switch to a non-toxic kitchen cleaner

Think Outside Your Workout Box How we exercise is as personal as the food we choose to eat. Just as it's important to listen to your body about which foods work best for you, you also need to listen to what your body tells you about your exercise. Whatever form of activity you enjoy, it should make your body feel great, physically and mentally, and you should not dread doing it (perhaps even look forward to it). At this point in the change process, it's a good time to ask yourself if you are continuing to do the same form of exercise out of pure habit? Think of the grandmother cutting the ends off the roast.

What are your personal fitness goals? Do you still get the same benefits from your exercise routine as you once did? Flexibility in your workout is just as important as your food flexibility. Just as your body needs a variety of fruits and vegetables, it also requires a variety of movement to stay healthy. Dare I say, at some point, you may also need to look at transitioning to some new forms of exercise that appreciate changes in your body. I'm not suggesting that you move from CrossFit six times a week to chair yoga, but I am suggesting that you take a step back and take an honest look at what your body needs physically and if your workout is still doing the trick.

I always say, if you don't like green smoothies then don't drink them. If you don't like running but do it every day because it's "good for you," then maybe you should look for other forms of cardio. Perhaps you would enjoy something else such as cycling, a row machine, or a brisk walk with your dog. It's okay to admit that you have outgrown your workout. It doesn't mean you are old or weak, but it does mean that it's important to respect your body. There are probably a lot of things that you used to do (and wear) in your younger days that you've outgrown. There are so many amazing workouts now and there is something for everyone at every age: power yoga, Buti yoga, barre3, Pilates, dance workouts, aqua cycling, hot Pilates, TRX, boxing, etc. Try something new and see how you feel. Trade free guest passes with your friends to try something new. Experiment with a variety of free online workouts that are outside of your typical exercise regimen. Practicing change in all aspects of your life, including your workout, is great for your mind and body!

I have seen variations of the following story many times.

> *Gwen is 54 and goes to a class every morning at 5:15am where she lifts heavy weights and does serious cross-training. She loves the class, but recently noticed that she has significant knee, back, and shoulder pain both during and after the class. She is also so tired and resists dozing off to sleep at her desk in the afternoon. She drinks coffee at 4 p.m. to get her through the dinner hour until she can crawl into bed as soon as the kids go to sleep. Perhaps a different form of exercise (or this one, but less often) would be kinder to her body, allow her to get a bit more sleep, and help Gwen stay strong.*

Here are a few questions to help you assess if it's time to change your workout:

> Do I look forward to exercising?

> Does my exercise give me energy throughout the day?

> Do I feel any pain during or after my workout?

> Does my exercise make me so tired that I can't function later in the day?

> Does my exercise give me the strength I need for daily life?

Inner Warrior I never realized how powerful a new form of exercise could be and how it can bring out your inner warrior! I recently found a new exercise that combines yoga, Pilates, and barre. It is challenging yet kind to my body. The workout provides a sense of calm and gives me strength both mentally and physically as well as creativity and inspiration (quite helpful when writing this book). When the music gets loud, the lights dim down and the workout gets tough, I feel an inner warrior emerge, and she looks like Wonder Woman's mother, with her sword and shield. I think of her strong body and determination to protect her child at all costs and prevent the dangers that lay ahead. I can totally relate to her. A few weeks after I began discovering my inner warrior, my husband came home with a surprise gift from a fundraising event. He won a beautiful necklace in the shape of a shield and now I wear it every day!

Who is the warrior that inspires you? Maybe it's your grandmother who raised her family as a widow, or your father who climbed out of poverty to create a better life, or a friend who has endured more hardship than anyone should have to bear. Channel that person in your workout and in your health journey and you will accomplish all your goals and way more.

Be Kind to Your Body When my health problems reached their peak, I was so determined to fix them that I tried everything. Body brushing, needles in my liver and tonsils, took over twenty supplements a day, and more. I was mad at my body for failing me. What I didn't realize was that my body was simply tired and had reached its limit of the amount of toxins, viruses, and stress that it could handle.

I began listening to a guided meditation before bed that targeted different health problems (back pain, digestion, stress, etc.). This was incredibly powerful as it allowed me to reflect on the specific problem I was dealing with and honor it. One night, I was listening to the topic of overall healing and I was physically startled by the woman's words, "Your body is doing the very best it can." Wow. It hit me and I immediately felt sad at how I was constantly beating my body up for failing me. It was only sending me signals that it needed help and couldn't function in the same mode anymore.

I began to picture an older man, perhaps my 86-year-old father, and imagined someone making him work or run really fast and getting angry at him for not keeping up. It was at that moment a real shift toward "kindness to my body" occurred.

I think of my own children when they are faced with too many stresses at school, sports, and with friends, and they start to act horribly. Perhaps all my body and my children need is some comfort and compassion. Be kind to your body, whether you are following a new food or wellness plan or trying a new workout. Today, I take time to thank and honor my body during my workouts and throughout the day. I am so grateful for health that sometimes it almost brings me to tears. While I still challenge myself, I do it carefully so no harm is done. Hopefully, my children will say the same thing.

Household/Beauty Supplies If you told me a few years ago that I would transition to a heavily plant-based, gluten-free, dairy-free food plan, that most of my household and beauty supplies would be non-toxic, and that my bras would no longer have underwire in them, I would have laughed in your face!

Honestly, I wasn't all that inspired to "clean up" my beauty or household products. I have always been a beauty product girl my whole life. A new lipstick or eyeshadow could pull me out of any bad day. As with perfecting a favorite recipe, it took me years to perfect a beauty regimen with all my favorite products from a variety of sources. However, I began to do some research on why this was so important to my health. Just a click, a documentary, and article away, I was shocked at the severe and detrimental effects of common cleaning supplies and popular weed killers on our health. Many metals, such as aluminum (found in everything from deodorant to antacids to cans), can build up and wreak havoc in our bodies. Apparently, everything in my house from my makeup drawer to my garage shelf was toxic. I was overwhelmed by it all, very similar to how I felt when faced with giving up my favorite foods.

There is a reason that it takes nine months to have a baby. We need the slow reminder each day that something big is going to happen and we need time to prepare. Imagine if you got pregnant and you had the baby in a week? That would be way too much change to handle. Think about changing your environmental products much the same way. Just as with your food transformation, do your research, talk to people you know, take baby steps, and use trial and error to slowly transition. Start with one or two things and slowly phase out existing products with non-toxic versions. Evaluate performance and cost to select the right products for you.

There are so many wonderful non-toxic beauty products out on the market today that do not include the carcinogens that are proven to cause cancer (or gluten for those with celiac). Natural products are a growing industry and there is a plethora of options for you to choose from. Even basic products like baking soda, vinegar, castile soap, and essential oils are quite effective in a variety of ways and making a huge comeback. Funny how change works. What's old is new again!

My waterproof mascara is the "last man standing" of beauty supplies. No matter how hard I try, I haven't found a replacement for the one I have used for many years. Maybe it is toxic, but I'm not going to cry about it, and if I did, you wouldn't see mascara running down my face.

Toxic Tribe The most important non-food that impacts your health is the tribe you surround yourself with. If you haven't already, get rid of toxic friends when you toss your toxic cleaning supplies (or at least move them to the back of the shelf). Your relationships with your tribe of family and friends cannot be purchased, they must be grown and cared for. Like a garden, you must pull the weeds to make room for those who mean the most. You also must fertilize the soil which means that no matter how long your "to-do" list is, a dinner out and a good laugh with those you care about is the best way to flourish.

Write and Burn We all have a lot of strong emotions that simply never see the light of day. We are all so busy that when you ask someone how they are doing, rarely do you get a real and honest response. God knows what would happen if every angry word from my head actually made its way to my mouth, especially to my children! I'm part Sicilian, after all, enough said.

If you have any unresolved issues or simply need to vent without consequences, try writing a letter and burning it. Be clear about your intentions. The idea is to release negativity, not get you riled up for an extended rant. This is your opportunity to say all the things you always wanted to say to one particular person or list of people. When it's time to burn your letter, mentally release all your pent-up emotions along with the ashes.

When I started thinking about this, I couldn't help but remember my great Aunt Ida. She had a mouth on her like a truck driver. She didn't need to write and burn because if she thought it, you heard it. She once was so mad at the popular bakery in the Italian section of South Philadelphia because she paid "good money" for a stale cake. They were not very receptive to this feedback and were, in fact, rude to her. BIG mistake. BIG. Like a bull in a china shop,

Aunt Ida walked down the center aisle of that store, cursing and waving her hands, knocking every pie, cake, and cookie tray off the displays lining the store. Talk about getting "whacked" in Philly—she was part of the pastry mob. But here's the thing about Aunt Ida: She was so funny and always had everybody around her laughing. She didn't pretend and certainly didn't hold in how she felt. She was strong as an ox and lived to be ninety-five. Maybe we can all learn a good lesson from her. I have to believe that there is a balance somewhere between "trashing the joint" and pretending all is "fine."

PERSONAL BITE

I experimented with the "write and burn" process and released so many emotions about a lot of things. Experts suggest cursing as a requirement for this exercise, so I unleashed my inner Aunt Ida and I can tell you pies were flying! It felt like a weight was lifted, like my soul was baptized again, and it felt great.

Stress and unspoken emotions can wreak havoc on your body when you least expect it. I never understood why a host of illnesses hit me when things were going just "fine." My friend and I joke that when you hear the phrase, "It's fine," you can rest assured that it's anything but.

This was never truer than when I was nine months pregnant. I was thrilled to be expecting my first child and beamed with delight, so why did I develop Bell's palsy then? The reality is that I was in denial about everything else happening in my life that was not so great. I moved back from Belgium because my grandmother died, I gained a ridiculous amount of weight, I went into preterm labor while my husband was still commuting to and from Germany, I was living in my parent's back bedroom because we couldn't find a house, and I was debating my future in management consulting. Now, I am not suggesting that I should have focused on all these negative things, but what I could have done was at least acknowledge them properly.

I'm proud to be a positive person and believe strongly in the power of positivity, but after several other battles with health problems throughout the last fifteen years (all while things were going "just fine"), I realized that it's okay to recognize, even honor, the things that suck in your life. "Write it and burn it" is a great way to do just that and keep moving forward.

BUSINESS BITE

When an organization stops looking ahead to change and improve, they stop period. Many strong businesses who have mastered a specific product choose to branch out into other product lines to expand their brand and increase sales. Take Ugg, for example, a very successful snow boot company. They have now launched into all sorts of clothing, loungewear, outerwear, and blankets (by the way, it is the most amazing blanket to curl up under and read a good book!). Just as businesses expand on a good product, you, too, must expand on your success and implement non-food changes as a way to push your health to the next level.

BEFORE YOU BITE

What non-food changes can you incorporate into your routine to create a true health transformation? Each year, we must take stock of our health to determine what changes are needed and what little steps can help get us there.

For example, your version of mindfulness might be as simple as turning the radio off when you drive for a little peace and quiet or you might simply take a minute to close your eyes and stretch at your desk. There are so many variations to choose from. You don't have to sit like a buddha for four hours to enjoy the effects of mindfulness. One practice you may want to try is setting a daily intention. Instead of rushing out of bed to grab your phone or get to work, consider placing your feet on the ground for sixty seconds and setting your intention for the day. This brief moment of time will give you the strength, focus, and purpose in facing the day ahead.

Go back and use your transition plan to make non-food changes to your life. Even something as small as taking the scenic path to work or school helps shift your thinking. As you have already learned with food, small changes can make a big difference in your health.

COMMUNICATION BITE

At the Institute for Integrative Nutrition, where I received my training, they taught us that all the broccoli in the world can't cure a bad relationship. This is a testament to the importance of all the non-food components of health. As you take yourself through The 5 Bites to Health, removing additional toxins from your body, don't forget to revisit and revise your health vision as you go. Challenge yourself to improve other factors in your health, such as the quality of your relationships, social life, spirituality and opportunities to demonstrate creativity. Think of each pass through the change model as simply another chapter in your health story. You will never stop changing and will hopefully continue adding chapters and volumes for years to come.

THE LAST BITE

Throughout this change process, I have grown so much more comfortable with my relationship between my body, my food, and my health. Like a marriage, we may get into an argument once in a while. If I don't take good care of myself and take my body for granted, it will fight back with a tingle or numbness in my leg, or in my face if it's a really big fight. But I know it's just my body's way of communicating, "I need you to pay more attention to me." This is sounding more like a marriage than I thought! I guess it all comes down to respect. If we respect each other, everything will stay cool!

We all have a health story to tell. I was lucky that mine didn't progress into something way worse, and I recognize that others' health problems are a lot more severe than mine. In gathering the data for the book, so many people opened up to share their personal stories of health, illness, and their journey to change in the hopes of helping others. I hope that through these stories and my five-step approach to change that more people will not only be inspired to change but now have the skills and tools to make it happen.

Looking back, I realize that I was always interested in health and wellness, but I had no idea that my eating habits weren't nearly as "healthy" as I thought. I wonder if I make a better health coach because I was a huge candy addict or in spite of it? I'm not a perfect eater even today and that's part of my plan for now. Truly fake food with an ingredient list a mile long is not something I am going to eat even if it is "only in moderation." But you will find me loving my apple with almond butter (maybe a couple dark chocolate mini chips) or my non-dairy yogurt with granola all day long.

I wish there were a silver bullet, one easy answer, or a quick pill for health. With so many people inspired to change but missing the toolkit to get there, I am so excited to share my experience in The 5 Bites to Health as a method for helping others in their own personal journey. Change is hard to digest sometimes. Trust the process, listen to your body, and you will be amazed. The answers were within all along.

ACKNOWLEDGMENTS

I am so grateful for my multi-talented husband for his constant support and encouragement, both in my own journey to health and throughout the book writing process. Thank you to my family and friends for listening to my stories of food, sensitivities, symptoms, toxins, and often unconventional wellness treatments without judgment. To my editor, Amanda, thank you for pushing me to stay authentic and for keeping me organized. To Amie and Sue, thank you for bringing my words to life in the cover and graphics. Ava, you are the best! Lauren and Joanna, thanks for your support literally every day from page one until the end.

To all the individuals I interviewed, to those who participated in the food transition survey, to my health coaching clients, and acquaintances along the way, thank you for sharing your personal struggles from illness to wellness. I am fascinated by your stories of discovery as you learned to interpret your body's secret language. Thanks for "spreading the love" with me.

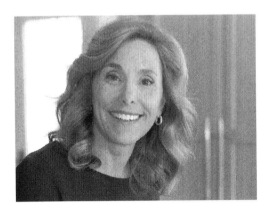

MEET THE AUTHOR

Marissa Costonis spent over ten years in Accenture's change management practice, leading a variety of change transformation initiatives around the world. After developing neuropathy and after a host of other health problems began to pile up, Marissa was faced with the challenge of fundamentally changing all her food and eating habits.

Overwhelmed and frustrated, Marissa began to apply all the leading change models to her own transformation. She discovered the secret to transitioning to a new way of eating was surprisingly hidden within the practices of successful organizations adept at change. Marissa decided to create a new change model that exposes the difficulties of change and supports the transition to health, one bite at a time.

Marissa graduated from the Institute for Integrative Nutrition and launched her health coaching practice, Change Bites, LLC. She conducts individual and group coaching programs, workshops, and enjoys guest speaking engagements to share her unique approach.

Marissa lives outside of Philadelphia with her husband and two children.

To share your own personal journey to health, for more information, or to contact Marissa visit: www.ChangeBites.com.

ENDNOTES

1. Tasler, Nick. "Stop Using the Excuse 'Organization Change is Hard.'" Harvard Business Review, 19 Dec. 2017, eld.hbr.org/2017/07/stop-using-the-excuse-organization-change-is-hard.

2. Wing R R & Jeffrey R. "Outpatient treatment of obesity: a comparison of methodology and clinical results." Int. J. Obesity 3:261-79, 1979.

3. "Autoimmune Info- American Autoimmune Related Diseases Association." AARDA, www.aarda.org/who-we-are/our-mission.

4. "Heart Disease and Stroke Statistics 2017 At-a-Glance." American Heart Association and American Stroke Association. 5 Jan. 2017.

5. JAMA Pediatrics. Study led by Jonathan Silverberg of St. Luke's-Roosevelt Hospital Center in New York.

6. Toole, Michelle "80% of Your Immune System is in Your GI tract." Healthy Holistic Living. http://www.healthy-holistic-living.com/probiotic-benefits.html

7. Miller, Sara G. "Here's How Many Heart Disease and Diabetes Deaths Are Linked to Food." Live Science, 7 Mar. 2017, 11:00am ET, www.livescience.com/58144-diet-death-heart-disease-stroke-diabetes.html.

8. Norton, Robert S. KaplinDavid P. "The Office of Strategy Management." Harvard Business review, 1 Aug. 2014, hbr.org/2005/10/the-office-of-strategy-management.

9. Gladwell, Malcolm, 1963. "The Tipping Point: How Little Things Can Make a Big Difference". Boston :Back Bay Books, 2002. Print.

10. "Netflix Says It Will Spend Up to $8 Billion on Content Next Year." The New York Times. 16 Oct. 2017 https://www.nytimes.com/2017/10/16/business/media/netflix-earnings.html

11. "Netflix Raised Prices and Still Signed up More Subscribers Than Ever Before." Quartz. 22 Jan. 2018. https://qz.com/1185744/netflix-raised-prices-and-more-people-signed-up-than-ever-in-q4-2017

12. "What Exactly Is Alternative Medicine?" WebMD, WebMD, www.webmd.com/balance/guide/what-is-alternative-medicine#1.

13. Nohria, Nitin, and Michael Beer. "Cracking the Code of Change." Harvard Business Review, 13 July 2015, hbr.org/2000/05/cracking-the-code-of-change.

14. "Does Self-Control Have a Limit?" Psychology Today, Sussex Publishers, www.psychologytoday.com/us/articles/201509/does-self-control-have-limit.

15. "Giving Thanks Can Make You Happier" Harvard Health Publishing, Harvard Medical School, Harvard Health Publishing https://www.health.harvard.edu/healthbeat/giving-thanks-can-make-you-happier

16. "The Sidur Sim Shalom, Prayer Book for Peace." The United Synagogue of Conservative Judaism, p. 149. 1998. Print.

ADDITIONAL RESOURCES
FOR HEALTH & CHANGE MANAGEMENT

....

Anderson, Dean, and Linda S. Ackerman-Anderson. *Beyond Change Management: Advanced Strategies for Today's Transformational Leaders.* San Francisco: Jossey-Bass/Pfeiffer, ©2001. Print.

Campbell, T. Colin, and Thomas M. Campbell II. *The China Study.* Dallas: BenBella Books, Inc., ©2004. Print.

Conner, Daryl. *Managing at the Speed of Change: How Resilient Managers Succeed and Prosper Where Others Fail.* Villard Books, ©1992. Print.

Duck, Jeanie Daniel. *The Change Monster.* Three Rivers Press, Inc. ©2001. Print.

Fuhrman, Joel. *Eat to Live.* Little, Brown and Company, ©2011. Print

HBR's 10 Must Reads on Change Management. Boston, Mass.: Harvard Business School Publishing Corporation, ©2011. Print.

Heath, Chip, and Heath, Dan. *Switch: How to Change Things When Change Is Hard.* Currency, ©2010. Print.

Hiatt, Jeff, and Timothy J. Creasey. *Change Management: The People Side of Change.* Prosci Inc., ©2012. Print.

Hyman, Mark. *The Blood Sugar Solution 10-day Detox Diet.* Little, Brown and Company/Hachette Book Group, ©2014. Print.

Kotter, J. P. *Leading Change.* Boston: Harvard Business School Press, ©2012. Print.

Pollan, Michael. *In Defense of Food.* The Penguin Group, ©2008. Print.

Pulde, Alona, and Lederman, Matthew. *Forks Over Knives Family.* Touchstone, ©2016. Print.

Rosenthal, Joshua. *Integrative Nutrition.* Greenleaf Book Group, ©2011. Print.

Seligman, Martin E.P. *Authentic Happiness: Using the New Positive Psychology to Realize Your Potential for Lasting Fulfillment.* Atria Paperback, ©2013. Print.